Die Fat or Get Tough

101 Differences in Thinking Between Fat People and Fit People

Steve Siebold

Die Fat or Get Tough

101 Differences in Thinking Between Fat People and Fit People

Steve Siebold

Published by
London House
www.londonhousepress.com

Ordering Information
To order additional copies, visit www.diefatbook.com
or by calling 561-733-9078

ISBN: 978-0-9755003-3-0

Credits

Editor: Brenda Robinson
www.potentpen.blogspot.com

Cover and Book design by Sandra A. Larson
www.SLDesignFX.net

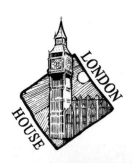

CONTENTS

Dedication

This book is dedicated to my wife of nearly 25 years, Dawn Andrews Siebold, the fearless leader of the Fat Loser Program. Your struggle and subsequent success in getting fit inspired me to write this book. You are my muse.

Thanks for being a role model to me and so many others. Thanks for being my friend and sharing your life with me.

I love you.

DIE FAT OR GET TOUGH

Introduction

Thank you for investing in this book. As clichéd as it sounds, I really believe it has the power to change your life. These concepts certainly changed mine.

For those of you who haven't read my first two books, *177 Mental Toughness Secrets of the World Class*; and *Coaching 177 Mental Toughness Secrets of the World Class*, I want to explain a couple of things. When I make reference to 'middle-class thinking or world-class thinking, I'm not referencing socioeconomic sub groups. Middle class in mental toughness language refers to the masses, while world class refers to the super-achievers. I use these references throughout all of my books to make the distinction in thinking, beliefs, philosophies and habits between the average person and the ultra successful. This may offend you, as it has other readers over the years, but it's impossible to dispute the huge gap between the haves and have nots. Instead of wasting your mental energy being offended, choose to think like the winners in life and join them in the victory lane.

This books hits hard and never lets up. All efforts to be politically correct were abandoned early in this project. There has been enough hand holding, wishful thinking and positive platitudes written on this topic to last forever. This book cuts through the delusional thinking of the masses with a machete and takes no prisoners. It will get you thinking about being fat in a way you may never have thought about it before. No matter how mentally tough you are, this book will send a lightning bolt of reality directly to your belief system. It will eliminate every excuse you've ever made for being fat. It will throw you up against the wall of objective reality and force you to see yourself as others see you. And when you emerge victorious, you will become a force of nature the likes of which very few people have ever experienced. You will begin to believe you can do anything…and you'll be right.

If at any time you fall into the middle class habit of looking for someone to blame, and you decide to attack me for being blunt, remember this: six years ago I was fat. I went from being a physical specimen who could run a 5 minute mile to fat tub-of-lard with my belly hanging over my belt. I was disgusted, so I got tough and fixed it. The information in this book comes from my own failure and subsequent success, as well as five years of research and interviews with hundreds of fat and fit people across the country. I know what it feels like to wake up in the morning, look in the mirror and get depressed. I lived it. I also know what it's like to win this fight, and exactly how you can do it, too.

I have good news and bad news about getting fit and healthy. The bad news is society has been lying to us for years. We've been told that getting fat is not our fault and it's easy to fix. We've been told diets don't work. We've even been coerced into believing big is beautiful. What's needed is a dose of objective reality, and since no one else seems willing to say it, I'm stepping up.

So here goes. You might want to sit down.

Being fat will make you sick. It will suck the energy out of your life. It will cost you money. It will damage your relationships. It will decimate your self esteem. Fat is deadly, ugly and unhealthy. But you already knew that, right? That's the bad news.

So what's the good news?

There's a solution. If you're ready to hear it.

Can you handle the truth?

Ok, here it is.

Unless you have a medical condition or psychological disorder, getting fat is your fault. It's not partly your fault; it's completely your fault. Food companies and restaurants might be making fat filled pizzas and burgers and serving them in larger portions, but you and I are the ones eating them. We're supposed to be mentally tough enough to walk away.

So what's the solution?

It's not easy, but it is simple.

Are you ready?

It's a two step process, and if you get it, you have a shot at living a long, healthy life with filled with boundless energy and world-class self confidence.

Step 1.   Consult your physician and select a world-class diet and exercise program.

Step 2.   Develop the mental toughness to stick to your diet and exercise program.

And that's it.

Die fat or get tough. Those are your options. It's that simple.

Now the choice is yours. Keep deluding yourself about what it really takes to get fit and healthy, or take responsibility for your habits, actions and behaviors and solve this life threatening problem once and for all.

I hope you decide to get fit and change your life forever. If you do, I promise it will be one of the most important things you ever do.

If you've ever wondered what you're made of, buckle your seat belt, because you're about to find out.

To your success!

Steve Siebold
February 3, 2009
Palm Beach, Florida

Acknowledgements

To **Dawn Andrews Siebold**, my wife, and head coach of the Fat Losers, for always believing in me and the mental toughness message, even when we were flat broke. I couldn't have done any of this without you.

To **Brenda Robinson**, my editor, for your ongoing guidance and ideas for this book. Your expertise and enthusiasm for this project was obvious from the beginning and very much appreciated.

To **Sandra Larson**, our graphic designer, for all of your hard work on the cover and layout of this book. You are a true professional.

To **Michael Altshuler**, the American Gladiator turned millionaire entre-preneur who served as my fitness role model. You're intensity and focus on fitness inspired me to get my old body back in 2003.

Fat people eat for pleasure

Fit people eat for health

The average person fortunate enough to live in a modern society with an abundance of food and the luxury of eating any time, views eating primarily as a pleasurable activity. Fit people see eating primarily as a means to increase health, energy and vitality. Food is viewed as a means to an end, rather than an end itself. While fat people are buying into advertising, connecting food with happiness, people who are thin and healthy ignore commercial propaganda and choose to educate themselves on the healthiest foods available. As a result of this vast difference in thinking and behavior, fat people eat for pleasure and create a never ending cycle of emotional addiction that accompanies an ever-expanding waistline. They experience nightmares about heart attacks, diabetes, and an overall loss of energy and stamina. Fit people choose to discipline themselves before they put anything in their mouth, and are able to enjoy what they eat without the guilt or fear of slowly destroying their own health. They know they will be healthier after a meal than they were before. Fat people expend more mental energy worrying about the aftereffects of poor food choices than fit people do in planning their diets. The thoughts that preoccupy the out of shape and obese segment of society are powered primarily by fear. These people are fat, but not stupid. They know they're slowly eating themselves to death, yet feel powerless to change. Meanwhile, fit people are eating merrily and celebrating a life of discipline, self-mastery, and abundant health. And the foundation of their success is eating for health instead of pleasure. This one small distinction in thinking can make the difference between world-class health and an early grave.

Critical Thinking Question

What are the three main reasons you eat when you're not hungry?

Action Step

For the next seven days, keep a written record of why you overeat and eat when you're not hungry, to see if patterns exist.

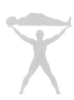

Fat people believe diets don't work

Fit people believe people don't work

A mericans have been programmed to believe diets don't work because of the inability of the average person to stick to them, and their unwillingness to take responsibility for their own failure. Make no mistake: many diets work very well. Because an individual lacks the mental toughness to stick to a diet doesn't make the diet any less effective. Fat people have a difficult time accepting responsibility for their own behavior, so they blame their diet. That's no different than a college graduate begging for money on the street and then blaming the school for his failure to succeed. This delusional thinking is a hallmark of the middle-class mindset. World-class thinkers know the real problem lies in the thoughts, beliefs and philosophies of the individual. They know diets work, but people often don't. Exacerbating the delusion of the masses are the weight loss companies telling people getting fat isn't their fault. Of course, this makes fat people feel comfortable with their failures, and comfort is the most important thing to the middle-class consciousness. So in addition to unhealthy foods, they begin ingesting pre-packaged meals and magical pills that promise to turn them into the next supermodel. To add insult to injury, these diet companies have the audacity to brainwash the masses into believing losing and maintaining their weight will be easy and effortless. Fortunately for these companies and unfortunately for their customers, fat people want to believe this so badly they lie to themselves. Human history is filled with examples of the masses willingly deceiving themselves into believing things that aren't true for the sake of psychological comfort. They lack the mental and emotional toughness to cope with objective reality. All this self- deception eventually leaves the person frustrated, unhappy and fatter than ever. At the same time this preventable tragedy is occurring, fit people are taking advantage of brilliant diets and getting superior results.

Fat Loser Quote

❝ *Make a decision to stop treating your diet like a hobby and start treating it like a battle you must win. Get tough and hold your feet to the fire. 99% compliance is failure. If you're going to get fit, it's all or nothing.* ❞

Critical Thinking Question

Have you bought into the middle-class belief that diets don't work?

Action Step

Start telling yourself you have 100% control over your own level of fitness.

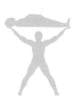

Fat people are waiting to be rescued from obesity

Fit people know no one is coming to the rescue

The middle-class mindset is famous for waiting for the hero on the white horse to rescue him from his problems. Whether it's their parents, the government, their spouse or the company they work for, many people have a deep rooted belief that it's someone else's responsibility to make them healthy, wealthy and happy. So when they get fat, not only do they blame the food companies and restaurants, they also expect something or someone to show up and save them from themselves. The great ones know if they get fat the only person who can save them is the man in the mirror. The mantra of the world world-class thinker has always been the same: I am responsible.

This is the cornerstone of their success in everything they do. If they need coaching, mentoring or support, they will ask for it without hesitation. The difference is no matter how much help they receive, they believe their success or failure is up to them. They refuse to blame anyone else for their shortcomings. If they lose focus and gain weight, you can bet it won't be long before they're back at their ideal weight, stronger than ever. Of course this is the general philosophy of world-class thinkers, so they are able to apply it in all areas of their lives. If you've ever wondered why some people seem to have it all, stop wondering and start dissecting their beliefs and philosophies on life and living. That's where their success begins.

Fat Loser Quote

Critical Thinking Question

Will this be the time you'll stick to your diet and succeed, or are you still waiting for the next magic pill, potion or program to save you?

Action Step

Accept full responsibility for getting fat, forgive yourself, and focus your mental energy on getting fit.

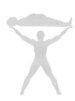

Fat people believe diets are fads

Fit people believe diets are strategies

The average person has been programmed to believe diets are short term fads designed for quick weight loss. World-class thinkers know a diet is a strategy designed to assist them in controlling their weight while enhancing their health, energy, and vitality. Fit people know their food intake must be systematically controlled and monitored for optimal results, and that it's an ongoing process that lasts a lifetime. The idea of randomly eating anything that's placed in front of them is a recipe for failure, frustration, and obesity. Like the rich man who monitors his money, fit people keep a close calculation of what they put into their mouth. In finance we call it a budget. In health, we call it a diet. Unfortunately, society has given diets a bad name by claiming they don't work. It's hard to deny the monetization of sickness. In essence, there's more money in helping people regain their health after they've systematically destroyed it than there is teaching them healthy prevention habits. I'm not blaming the health care profiteers for capitalizing on the predictability of human behavior. Their responsibility is to their shareholders, not us. That's capitalism. What I'm saying is, it's our job to recognize the inherent conflict of interest involved in the health care industry that most people count on to save them.

Fat Loser Quote

❝ *Fit people love to eat the same foods as fat people, but they choose health over gluttony. Their fitness is the result of a calculated strategy.* ❞

Critical Thinking Question

Do you see your diet as a brilliant strategy, or a daily burden?

Action Step

Write down the three biggest lies that are perpetuated by the masses, the media, and the health care industry out of deceit or delusion.

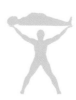

Fat people eat emotionally

Fit people eat strategically

One of the primary reasons middle-class thinking leads to obesity is emotional eating. When fat people feel bad, they eat. When they're happy, they eat. For the average person, eating is a way to enhance pleasure and ease pain. Food is used as a drug to alter unpleasant moods, and this behavior is a habit some people carry with them from childhood to old age. What makes this habit worse is, the good feelings food produces are short lived, which means you have to keep eating to continue experiencing pleasure. This is one of the reasons people stuff themselves at mealtimes. Fit people avoid emotional eating, choosing to eat only when hungry. They use logic instead of emotion to dictate and control their food intake, and are acutely aware of the tendency to use food as a drug. It's not that they're not tempted to eat emotionally; it's that they put logical thinking ahead of emotional thinking. The secret to their success is awareness, planning, and critical thinking. They've learned to control their emotions by recognizing habitual triggers that lead to unhealthy choices. Middle-class thinking says eat whenever you get hungry or when it feels good. World-class thinking says eat when you get hungry; and eat strategically for maximum energy, vitality and strength. Fat people are controlled by their emotions. Fit people exercise emotional control in everything they do.

Fat Loser Quote

❝ Mental Toughness means learning to control your emotions. People with middle-class consciousness get inconsistent results because they are slaves to their emotions. This is the psychological makeup of the yo-yo dieter. ❞

Critical Thinking Question

What are your three most powerful emotional eating triggers?

Action Step

The next time you reach for food out of pure emotion, put the food down and walk away. Begin to question your psychological motives every time you eat.

Fat people give into cravings

Fit people prepare for cravings

Cravings are one of the most common downfalls of the average dieter. Since most people never make a serious commitment to getting thin and healthy, cravings are a real threat. The problem with giving in to cravings is allowing old eating habits to creep back into your life and threaten to take you back to where you began. Fit people know giving into cravings, no matter how small, is a slippery slope and a dieting disaster. Fat people fall into this trap because they haven't made a serious commitment to reach their ideal weight. Middle-class thinking tells the person this little cheat meal won't make that big of a difference, and besides, you can always start over again on Monday. These people treat dieting like a hobby instead of a major behavioral change. The problem is that any solid diet requires strict compliance to work, especially in the beginning. To fit people, cravings are a challenge and a litmus test rolled into one. Dieting when you're full is easy. Sticking to your diet when you're hungry takes courage. The media and so-called experts claim successful dieting isn't about willpower. This is like saying war isn't about violence. It's a nice idea, but not an actual fact. The truth is any major discipline or accomplishment requires substantial willpower in the early stages. Later on, your new eating habits will ease your desire for unhealthy foods. But the truth is, no matter how long you maintain your weight; you will always have to be on guard against slipping back into old habits. This is the glamourless reality experts only discuss among each other, because they know most people can't handle the truth.

Fat Loser Quote

    66 *Periodic cravings are like pop quizzes thrown at you randomly to test your commitment to your diet. Pass enough pop quizzes and your grade is guaranteed. Tough out enough cravings and your fitness is guaranteed.* 99

Critical Thinking Question

Are you adequately prepared for all the obstacles you will face on the road to fitness?

Action Step

Identify your most powerful craving and a meal, snack or dessert on your diet that will satisfy it.

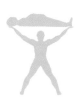

Fat people are controlled by food

Fit people are guided by vision

Fat people are at the mercy of their hunger, cravings, and eating habits. Breakfast, lunch, and dinner dominate their daily planning, though most of them are not consciously aware of it. After years of being controlled by food, they develop the belief that they are powerless in this area. This damages their self-esteem and bleeds over into other areas of their lives. Fit people have the opposite experience. Since they've mastered the eating/thinking equation, they believe they have the power to accomplish anything they set their mind to. In a country where being fat and out of control is the norm, being thin, healthy and responsible creates a tidal wave of self-confidence that has a positive impact on everything the person touches. That's why so many world-class thinkers become great visionaries: the confidence gained through success expands their consciousness and solidifies the belief they have the power to do anything. This confidence leads them to behave in ways that support their belief, which ultimately leads them to greater success. Their success becomes a self-fulfilling prophecy that all begins with self-control. Once their emotionally charged visions are in place, the belief they have in themselves to make it reality drives them to take action, again and again.

Fat Loser Quote

" The 'how to' of weight loss is simple. There are hundreds of diets created by brilliant doctors all over the world. The challenge in losing and maintaining weight isn't the how, it's the why. It's not enough to know how to do something. You must know exactly why you are doing it. Why will you fight? Why will you suffer through this process? If you don't have a compelling reason for losing weight, you're going to be emotionally vulnerable when the going gets tough. "

Critical Thinking Question

Do you have a crystal clear vision of what your life will be like as a fit person?

Action Step

Put your vision on paper and describe what it feels like to be a fit person as though it's already happened.

Fat people believe there's a hidden secret to being healthy

Fit people know there is no secret

One of the hallmarks of middle-class thinking is the idea there are shortcuts and secrets to success. What it takes to become and stay thin and healthy has been known for many years: making a decision to begin a healthy diet and exercise program, and developing the mental toughness to stick with it. That's it. That's always been it. There's nothing mysterious about losing weight. There's nothing mysterious about maintaining weight. Instead of searching for the latest diet, fit people focus on staying mentally tough and disciplined. They work on changing the way they see eating and exercise while they reprogram their beliefs about what tastes and feels good. They learn to ignore the messages sold to the public about dieting. They come to terms with the fact that losing and maintaining weight is simple, but not easy. They realize their willpower is the only thing standing between them and the body they want. Instead of wasting mental energy scheming for an easier way to win the battle of the bulge, they make a commitment to make their health and fitness goals a reality and go to work to achieve it. While fat people are jumping from diet to diet, fit people are basking in the glory of their success. Their laser focus on the real "secret" of weight loss leads them to a quick and decisive victory, which gives them time to focus the same organized concentration on their next goal.

Fat Loser Quote

❝ *Fat people get fit by staying compliant with their diet. Period. There is no secret. Yes, you have to be mentally tough to be compliant, but there is no mystery. People who stay compliant get fit, and people who don't die fat. Stop wasting time looking for an easier way. Just stick to the diet and get it over with.* ❞

Critical Thinking Question

Do you believe there's a secret to getting fit, or is the real secret just plain old discipline, willpower and hard work?

Action Step

Just for today, decide to be mentally tough and stick to your diet and exercise plan.

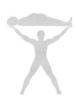

Fat people are afraid of being fat

Fit people aren't afraid of anything

The average person has been psychologically conditioned to operate from a fear and scarcity consciousness. This programming begins in childhood and is reinforced throughout most people's lives. . .unless they have exposure to world-class thinking strong enough to break the cycle of fear. This is a rare occurrence. Weight loss is no exception. Middle-class thinking attaches fear to everything, and the more someone fears being fat the more likely it will happen. World-class thinking is rooted in love and abundance, which is always moving the person toward his goals and dreams as opposed to moving away from fear. Fit people set ultra specific health and fitness goals, and spend their mental energy moving toward them. Since fear based thinking rarely enters their minds, they immediately begin moving forward like a locomotive thundering down the track devoid of the psychological interferences that plague most people. While the masses waste their mental energy in fear-based thinking, the great ones bathe in thoughts of love, abundance and gratitude. Every thought moves them closer to their ultimate vision. When it comes to dietary choices, fat people focus on the fear of missing out on eating the foods they love. Fit people condition themselves to focus on the foods that move them toward their ideal weight. The masses focus on the foods they've lost. Champions focus on the foods they have. It's a distinction that makes the difference between failure and success.

Critical Thinking Question

What role has fear
played in keeping you fat?

Action Step

Start to notice when you begin thinking
fear based thoughts and ask yourself—does
this serve my own best interests?

Fat people expect weight loss without pain

Fit people know know everything has a price

Psychological delusion tells the middle-class thinker to expect world-class results from a middle-class effort. This is why most people go on and off diets their entire lives. The premise in thinking is simple: discover a painless diet that doesn't require discipline or sacrifice. Of course this diet doesn't exist, but advertisers are shrewd enough to know they can easily fool the masses into believing it does. Not because the masses are stupid, but because they want the easy diet so badly they'll believe anything. It's like selling water to a man crawling through the desert. By the time he figures out it's not water, he's emptied the bottle. This snake oil salesmanship has been around since the beginning of time. Whether it's an easy diet, get-rich-quick scheme, or a surefire way to get to heaven, people of influence have always controlled the self-delusional thinking of the masses. If it feels good, sounds sweet and looks easy, right brain emotional thinking often overcomes left brain logic. The proof is in the success of advertisers and marketers. They get richer while the masses get fatter. The trap is easy to fall into, but the truth is simple: if you want to become thin and healthy, you will pay a price. You will sacrifice and call on every ounce of willpower you have. Once you reach your ideal weight, you will have to be on high alert every day of your life in order to not fall back into your old, well established habits. If you let your guard down, you'll be fat again. If you don't, you won't. The choice is yours. Pay the price for success, or pay the price of regret. But either way, rest assured, you will pay a price.

Critical Thinking Question

Do you believe your path to fitness is going to be pain free?

Action Step

Mentally prepare yourself for the struggle that often accompanies any major change in habits.

Fat people are delusional about being fat

Fit people operate from objective reality

Since human beings are emotional creatures, staying grounded in objective reality requires effort. It's easy to look in the mirror and not see what the world sees. The emotional brain protects us from pain by clouding the picture. There are ways around this phenomenon, however. When we see a photograph of ourselves, it seems to cut through the delusion and allows us to see what we really look like. Fit people use tools like this to keep themselves on track. One of the strategies we use in our Fat Losers program is to have people carry around a five pound bag. It doesn't sound like a lot of weight, but after you carry it around all day you begin to get an idea of the added strain your body experiences with a little extra weight. Another tool to keep you in objective reality is to ask people who care to tell you when you looked the best in your life. Chances are they will say when you were thinner. This negates the notion that our friends and family don't see the difference in our weight. They do, but out of kindness, they don't tell us. This can be deadly. Fat robs you of energy, vitality, and enthusiasm. It may even kill you. There's nothing good about it. The 'feel good' marketing scheme that says "big is beautiful" and people should be happy with their body no matter how fat they are, is a twisted lie. Fat sucks the life out of people. End of story. The choice is simple: DIE FAT OR GET TOUGH.

Fat Loser Quote

"The middle-class consciousness uses terms like overweight, heavy, big boned, and pleasingly plump to describe themselves and other fat people. This delusion makes them feel comfortable with their failure to control their body. The world class deal from objective reality and describe themselves as fat. The delusional approach gives the person permission to continue eating, while the objective reality method causes enough emotional pain to stop the destructive behavior."

Critical Thinking Question

If objective reality is on one end of the spectrum and self-delusion on the other, where does your thinking about fat and fitness fall most of the time?

Action Step

Just for today, decide to operate from 100% objective reality around your diet and exercise program. Refuse to allow delusional thoughts to cloud your judgment.

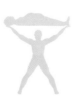

Fat people see food as their enemy

Fit people see food as their friend

Average people approach a diet as though they're being forced to give up foods they love. They see healthy foods as their enemy. Fit people have the opposite belief. They see healthy foods as friends that will help them achieve their ultimate physique. While the masses are avoiding their enemy, the classes are embracing their newfound friend. This distinction in thinking has a major impact on how the person feels about his diet, as well as how long he sustains new eating habits. This affects attitude and enthusiasm, which must remain strong, especially in the beginning and during periods of weight loss plateaus. Outside the physical component of eating, successful dieting is all mental toughness. It's not that you have to be perfect to succeed, but be aware that little things add up. One middle-class thought is no big deal, unless it leads to another. It's no different on the physical plane: eating one doughnut isn't the problem; it's what it leads to that makes it dangerous. Middle-class thinking is a slippery slope that leads most people into an unhealthy pattern of thought. It's easy to fall into, because it's the thinking of the majority of people. Is it any wonder so many people are overweight and out of shape? In actual fact, it's very predictable, and it will continue. But that doesn't mean you can't break out. It only requires a decision and the mental toughness to stick to it. Healthy food and exercise are friends that never let you down. No one is trying to take away the foods you love, nor is food your enemy. It's all in the way you decide to perceive it.

Fat Loser Quote

“ *The human brain's primary purpose is the preservation of the mind and body. When an event occurs, the brain asks three questions: 1. What is it? 2. What does it mean? 3. What do I do? If you can reframe the meaning of the event, you can alter the response that's sent back from the brain. Example: The event is someone offering you a hot fudge sundae. You interpret the sundae as something that will give you massive pleasure. As a result, you eat it. All you have to do is change what the sundae represents and you will change your behavior. If the sundae means you're on your way to getting even fatter and unhealthier, you will not eat the sundae. Representations are one of the secrets of successful behavior change.* ”

Critical Thinking Question

Are you cursing and complaining about
eating the foods and doing the exercises
that will make you fit and healthy?

Action Step

Start talking about your new food choices
and exercise habits as though they're
your new best friends that are going to
help you live a happier, healthier life.

Fat people believe obesity won't kill you

Fit people believe obesity won't kill you tomorrow

Many people who are more than fifty pounds overweight actually believe they are in no physical danger. Some doctors are even telling obese patients they are healthy. With all the information available on the threats of obesity, this is a classic example of self-delusion. Fit people believe fat might not kill you tomorrow, but it will probably kill you eventually. Along the way is type two diabetes and a vast array of ailments that will rob you of energy, health and happiness. These long term effects are easy for the masses to ignore because they don't appear immediately. This is often referred to as "whistling past the graveyard." No matter how you label it, the facts are the same: obesity will make you sick. . .eventually. One way or another, you're going to pay the price for being fat. It may not be today or tomorrow, but odds are, the longer you're fat, the more likely you will suffer catastrophically. Fit people know the battle of the bulge is a war that must be won. The older you are, the more important it is. Health and fitness cannot be purchased or won by political favor. It must be earned the old fashioned way: through hard work, discipline and willpower. Whatever you hear to the contrary is a lie. The good news is the benefits of winning the weight war outnumber the cost of success. Not only are you going to live longer and stronger, your success is going to positively impact every area of your life and influence the people around you.

Critical Thinking Question

Do you really understand how dangerous being fat is? Do you really understand how much energy, vitality and life is being sucked out of you to support all the excess fat you're carrying around?

Action Step

Write down three ways fat kills people or shortens their lives.

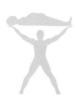

Fat people make excuses for being fat

Fit people know there is no excuse

Middle-class thinking is mired in excuses: tough childhood, bad parents, lousy teachers, overbearing religious leaders, heartless coaches, etc. The masses love to play the blame game, especially when it comes to dieting. They say diets don't work, which is reinforced by the organizations that benefit by perpetuating this lie. They surround themselves with people who believe the lie as much as they do, and together they eat their way into mediocrity and self-destruction. Fit people owe their success to a mindset of self-reliance and personal responsibility. The great ones grow up emotionally and realize the majority of the population never evolves past the limiting programming they received as children, and that the only way to break out is through adopting new beliefs and philosophies that serve their best interests. There is no excuse for being fat. The only logical option is to get thin and healthy by refusing to let yourself off the hook. Champions use their mental energy to create the body they desire, and they tap their mental toughness reservoir to help them stick to it. Once they start the diet, they refuse to look back. Their whole focus is manifesting the picture of the body they want on the movie screen of their mind, and any mental backtracking or breakdown is unacceptable. If they happen to mentally slip for even a second, they refocus immediately. World-class thinkers are much harder on themselves than any outside person has a right to be. This hardcore approach eliminates the struggle of yo-yo dieting and excuse laden performance.

Critical Thinking Question

What was the excuse you gave yourself
and others for failing on your last diet?

Action Step

Decide today that this time you're on a no excuses
diet. Fat losers don't make excuses, but losers do.

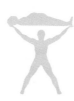

Fat people believe you get fatter as you age

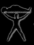

Fit people believe you have to be more strategic as you age

It may be harder to lose and maintain weight as you get older, but that just means becoming more strategic. The masses use age as another excuse for having a bloated, fat, unhealthy body; it's widely accepted by the middle-class as an irreversible fact. The truth is, with mental toughness you can be thin and healthy at any age, if you're tough enough to keep your commitment. Age is simply one more variable to factor into your weight loss and maintenance equation. While fat people are telling themselves and others their weight gain is the result of age and not their fault, fit people are firmly grounded in objective reality. They know you can get fat at any age if you're not eating consciously. That's why so many kids are fat. They're wolfing down doughnuts and French fries and mainstream society is saying its ok and encouraging them to be happy with their bodies, no matter how unhealthy they are. Champions are disgusted by this middle-class brainwashing administered by well meaning, unaware people. Strategic thinking and planning is critical to your weight loss/maintenance success, no matter how old or young you are. A little strategy goes a long way, and many diets are very thorough. You don't even have to create the strategy; all you have to do is follow it. The older you get, the more important maintaining a healthy weight becomes. The harder your body has to work, the less energy and vitality you'll have left to live the life you desire. Think strategically and never allow yourself an inch for excuses.

Critical Thinking Question

Do you really believe you're
fat because you're old?

Action Step

Start to challenge the beliefs and
philosophies of the mediocre masses,
especially in the area of health and fitness.
This is what keeps them mediocre.

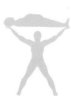

Fat people
see exercise as a chore

Fit people see exercise as fun

In the age of video games, remote controls and ultra modern conveniences, the masses see movement and physical effort as work. Society has been conditioned by advertisers to believe a sedentary lifestyle equals luxury. The idea of exercise for the sake of physical and mental fitness is beyond the belief system of most middle-class thinkers. In the linear mindset of the average person, exercise means expending energy they don't have. World-class thinkers know the nonlinear nature of exercise means the more energy you expend, the more you get back and the greater your stamina becomes. Fit people see exercise the same way they see other mandatory habits such as brushing teeth, showering, and eating a healthy diet. It's not that they have more discipline than fat people, they simply have different beliefs. Physically fit people possess a set of beliefs that drive them to place a high value on exercise. Some of them enjoy it more than others, but all of them share the belief that regular exercise is a non-negotiable habit that must be established and maintained for life. So while the masses are avoiding exercise at all costs, fit people are joining health clubs and investing in fitness equipment in record numbers. One group gets fatter and unhealthier every year, while the other continues to thrive and get stronger. The only difference between the two extremes is what they choose to believe about exercise.

Critical Thinking Question

Have you committed to make exercise one of your primary daily habits?

Action Step

Decide right now how much time you will invest exercising each day, and place as much importance on it in your daily routine as going to work.

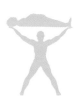

Fat people expect results without change

Fit people expect results through personal growth

Fat people believe the thinking that got them fat will make them thin. They believe they can play with their diet like a toy, and then blame the diet when they fail to lose weight. When they sit down to watch hours of television or surf the web every night, they feel validated when advertisers assure them diets don't work and it's not their fault they're fat. They refuse to change, yet they expect to miraculously lose weight. Fit people know all real change starts with the personal growth of the individual combined with the desire to get better results. They know advertisers say what people want to hear so they can sell products. Great performers are self-reliant and refuse to buy into the Madison Avenue propaganda. With their feet firmly planted in objective reality, they realize they are the problem and the solution. When they make a decision to change, they do it quickly and rarely look back. While the masses are easily knocked off course, the world class builds a protective cocoon around themselves to ward off temptation and stay laser focused on their objective. Once they make a decision to change their thinking, they let go of the past and focus on the beautiful future that awaits them at their ideal weight. To assist them in the process, they will often seek coaching or mentoring that includes a support system to help them accelerate their personal growth. While the masses like to laugh and scoff at the self-help movement, the great ones ignore them and get all the help they can. Once the change is made and the eating/exercise war is won, fit people continue to stand guard to be sure the old habits never return.

Fat Loser Quote

66 *Weight loss and control is about changing the thoughts, feelings and attitudes that govern your eating and exercise regimen. While most people evolve slowly and rarely challenge their own limiting beliefs, the great ones are growing every day by tapping into people operating at a higher level of consciousness. Passion for personal growth is one of the hallmarks of the world class.* 99

Critical Thinking Question

Have you committed to an ongoing program of personal growth?

Action Step

Make personal growth books, recordings and seminars a part of your daily life and watch your results skyrocket. (Less than 5% of the population does this.)

Fat people believe they can always start over on Monday

Fit people know Monday is never coming

Narcotics are the scourge of the poverty class. Alcohol is a killer of the working class. Self-delusion is the addiction of the middle class. While fat people delude themselves into believing they can continue starting over on Monday and eventually succeed, critical thinkers recognize this common psychological trap. The core belief is "I can eat the same and get different results". Fit people force themselves to grow up emotionally and take control of their minds and bodies. A fat person on a diet who is only semi-committed to success is no different than a school kid who refuses to concentrate on his/her homework, or a child who goes kicking and screaming at the first sign of having to exert self-control. Uncommitted dieters will use every self-deluding tool in the book to justify their lack of discipline and self-control. With the majority of the media and advertisers supporting their belief that diets don't work, they feel vindicated and go right back to eating like a fat person. Critical thinkers know that saying diets don't work is like saying exercise doesn't work. It's a ridiculous claim that's perpetuated for the purpose of manipulating the masses to buy the latest pill, potion or wonder drug that will make them thin and healthy. So the masses feel comfortable while they eat themselves into an early grave, and the producers of the cure-alls laugh all the way to the bank. It's pathetic and borderline criminal. The fact is, we are all responsible for our own decisions, mindsets, and even our diet and exercise programs. If the masses are foolish enough to believe every advertiser has their best interests at heart, they're going to be manipulated their entire lives. Critical thinkers take full responsibility for their results, and rarely believe profit driven claims that make the difficult appear easy. Starting over (again) Monday is an endless loop that keeps people fat forever.

Fat Loser Quote

When you're tempted to cheat, ask yourself these questions: when am I going to stop starting over? What makes tomorrow better than today to get fit? If I continue starting over every time the going gets tough, will I eventually die fat?

Critical Thinking Question

Have you fallen into the 'start over on Monday' trap?

Action Step

Wake up and realize Monday is never coming. Today is the day to start down the road to better health and fitness.

Fat people are motivated by fear and scarcity

Fit people are motivated by love and abundance

Fat people usually decide to lose weight when the fear of not doing so exceeds their fear of not being able to gorge on their favorite foods. The mindset of the masses is rooted heavily in fear and scarcity beginning in childhood, and the strongest fear becomes the biggest motivator. Fear is the bully that keeps the middle class handing over their lunch money and being grateful things aren't worse. The middle-class thinker sees happiness as the absence of pain. World-class thinkers are driven by the promise of a better life, and rarely allow fear to dictate their behavior. The great ones create a vision and take action to build legs under the picture in their minds. They wake up one day and realize they could be thinner and healthier, and then systematically move toward a life of healthy eating and robust exercise. Every day of their new routine moves them closer to the beautiful vision they have of a well-sculpted, energy abundant body that looks good and feels great. So while the middle class is running from one fear to satisfy another, the world class is moving toward a life most people only see in movies. They build massive momentum by imagining themselves at their perfect weight. They go to bed at night dreaming of the day they hit the magic number and imagine how it will feel to succeed in an area of life where most people fail. As their psychological momentum builds and they get closer to their dream, their level of excitement and enthusiasm begins to affect every other area of their lives. They eventually realize that moving toward a goal through love and abundance is the secret to success in every aspect of life. The result is a world-class performer who is thin, healthy, and on her way to the same success in any area she sets her sights on.

Critical Thinking Question

Are you motivated more by the pain of being fat or the pleasure of being fit? Is this helping or hurting you?

Action Step

Just for today, become hyperconscious of the state of mind that drives your behavior to determine if you're more motivated by fear and scarcity or love and abundance.

DIE FAT OR GET TOUGH

Fat people believe weight loss is complex

Fit people believe weight loss is simple

Fat people have failed on so many diets they begin to believe there's something mysteriously complex about getting thin and healthy. It's a psychological phenomenon that holds people back from building the body they desire and deserve. Fit people know weight loss is as simple and straightforward as making a commitment to change and being mentally tough enough to stick to their commitment. The configuration of the diets themselves can be very complex, but adhering to a diet is as elementary as having the willpower to keep your word to yourself. Fat people have no credibility with themselves because they've broken their own promises so many times they no longer trust their ability to do what they say they will do. This bleeds over into every area of their lives and destroys their self-esteem. Fit people make a decision and stick to their diet no matter how much they are tempted and taunted by themselves or others. They know being physically fit goes beyond looking good and being healthy. It impacts everything they do. The masses love to make the simple seem complicated so they have an excuse for failing. Champions keep it simple and get busy getting what they want. Instead of wasting their mental energy going from diet to diet, they select a diet and focus on following it to the letter until they arrive at their ideal weight. While fat people are struggling at every meal deciding whether or not to remain compliant, fit people waste no mental energy because the decision has already been made.

Critical Thinking Question

Do you realize how simple getting thin and healthy really is, or are you still trapped in middle-class thinking?

Action Step

Make the distinction in your thinking between something simple and something easy. Fitness is simple but not easy. Math is easy but not simple. This clarification helps you focus your efforts where they are needed most.

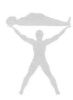

Fat people see exercise as a burden

Fit people see exercise as a privilege

Fat people view exercise as drudgery they neither enjoy nor place any value on. The idea of sweating and working out strikes them as a waste of time and energy. Fit people know exercise is one of the most important habits anyone can develop. They either love it or they don't, but either way they discipline themselves, knowing it's a non-negotiable practice. They know the benefits of physical exercise go far beyond losing and maintaining weight. Daily workouts sharpen their mental faculties, and many people claim it has a spiritual effect on them. Fit people see recreational exercise as a privilege only a small percentage of the world's population is fortunate enough to enjoy. They are grateful for the opportunity and take full advantage of their prosperity and good fortune. While fat people are complaining about having to exercise, fit people are happily working out and basking in thoughts of gratitude as they get stronger and healthier. Not only do they get the benefits of exercise, they also build the world-class habit of immersing their consciousness in thoughts of love, abundance and gratitude. This is one of the hallmarks of world-class thinking, and it carries over into every aspect of their lives. Once they experience the power of this positive psychological tidal wave they develop even more reverence for the act of physical exercise. Missing even one day of exercise, to a fit person is a big deal. They feel physically, mentally and spiritually sluggish without it. This is why they go to great lengths to maintain their workout routines when they travel, during holidays or in the event of any other inconvenient obstacle. They see it as a daily habit that cannot be missed.

Fat Loser Quote

“ Build this world-class belief: ‘I enjoy exercising because it makes me feel great.’ Program this belief even if you hate exercising, and after a few weeks you will begin to notice a subtle shift in your attitude towards exercise. ”

Critical Thinking Question

Do you believe exercise is a
privilege or a burden?

Action Step

Examine your core beliefs about exercise
and ask yourself if they are dictating
behaviors that are in your best interests.
Modify, change or eliminate any beliefs that
are leading you to middle-class results.

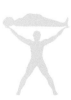

Fat people want an easy diet

Fit people want an effective diet

Unsuccessful people in any area of life are famous for looking for shortcuts to success. Whether it's getting rich, building relationships or losing weight, they're in the habit of directing their mental energy toward an easier way instead of an effective way. This is classic middle-class thinking, and it's created the fattest population in the world. Fit people are grounded in objective reality. They expect to pay a price for success and focus all their energy on building and maintaining the necessary habits required for success. This is true of world-class thinkers in general. While the masses are in a perpetual state of on again-off again decision making, the great ones rarely reverse major decisions. They ignore the middle-class programming of the masses and elect to follow world-class thinkers more successful than themselves. This is the reason the rich get richer, the fit, fitter, the healthy relationships, healthier, etc. It's not about food or exercise. It's about how these two groups think about food and exercise. Our beliefs about anything dictate our behavior towards it. The most effective way to get fit is to identify your beliefs about diet and exercise and ask yourself if they're helping or hurting you, and make adjustments as necessary. Fit people know effective thinking is just as important as following an effective diet.

Fat Loser Quote

❝ There are no shortcuts to dieting. You either adhere to a healthy diet or pay the price of sickness and disease. Looking for quick fixes is a habit that must be broken if you're going to be fit. Remember that this is not a short term project. This is a lifetime process that only ends when they haul you off to the graveyard in a pine box. Until that day, fitness is essential and must be approached like any other long term investment. ❞

Critical Thinking Question

Are you on a diet that's easy or effective?
Can you stay on this diet long term?

Action Step

Stop looking for an easy diet. Realize that any major habit change will be moderately to very difficult for the first 21-30 days. Get on a solid diet your physician recommends and stay mentally tough until it gets easier.

Fat people see diets as short term

Fit people see diets as long term

Society has us programmed to believe diets are short term by nature, and that long term adherence to a healthy diet is impossible. This absurdity is perpetuated by people who have something to gain by giving fat people an excuse for failing in the dieting process. This idea has become so pervasive that even many dieting experts have bought into it. The masses have been systematically brainwashed to believe altering what you eat is impossible. Common sense tells us any habit can be changed, but the failure rate among dieters is so high that something or someone has to be blamed. Since most people can't come to terms with the reality that they're fat as a result of their own mental weakness and poor habits, they happily buy into the idea that diets don't work long term. Fit people are emotionally mature enough to see life as it actually is, instead of how they wish it was. They choose a diet they can stay on for life that serves them and makes them healthier. The concept of short term dieting is as ridiculous to them as short term exercising. Why start a diet or exercise program you can't stick to? It's like quitting smoking for a month knowing you're going to start up again. The only way this grade school level lie can be sold to millions of intelligent people is through the smokescreen of feel-good delusion. Fat people need to believe failing is not their fault, so they close their eyes and allow themselves to be manipulated by the profiteers of the weight loss industry. Meanwhile, fit people are happily enjoying the long term benefits of a world-class diet and exercise program.

Fat Loser Quote

❝ Succeeding on your diet in the long term will serve as an ongoing touchstone of achievement in your life. You'll always be able to draw on your fitness success as a confidence builder when you're approaching new challenges in your life, and no one will ever be able to take it away from you. Do you really understand how deep this goes? ❞

Critical Thinking Question

Do you see your new eating and exercise habits as short or long term?

Action Step

Start thinking of your health and fitness goals as something you're going to do for a lifetime. Avoid fad diets that last 30 days and magic pills that claim to make fat disappear. Invest 21-30 days of mental toughness into habits that will last a lifetime. Every time you make a major change, you must go through the 21-30 day period. Decide to do it one time and get it over with.

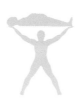

Fat people are erratic dieters

Fit people are consistent dieters

Middle-class thinkers are erratic, especially with anything requiring effort and discipline. World-class thinkers know erratic behavior in anything is a losing game, and this includes dieting. Fat people approach dieting like a hobby. Fit people approach dieting like a war. They overtake the bad habits and bring in new ones, and then stand guard when the old habits attempt to return. The great ones know consistency is the mark of the pro in any endeavor, so they consistently follow their diet and make food choices in their long term best interests instead of their short term cravings. The lack of consistency among the masses is so well documented that entire industries are based on the premise that only a small percentage of people will finish what they start. Health clubs oversell memberships by large numbers because they know most people will quit within 30 days. It's not working out that causes them to quit, it's the mindset of the quitter. Quitting is a habit. Fortunately, so is consistency. Everyone who chooses to can break the cycle of erratic performance by changing the way they think about it. Society was responsible for programming us as children, but we are responsible for changing our thinking to serve our own best interests. Consistency is a must-have quality for anyone who wants to be fit.

Fat Loser Quote

66 *Lasting behavior change requires that you ascend to a higher level of consciousness than you were operating from when you got fat. Albert Einstein said it best: 'A problem cannot be solved at the same level in which it occurred.' Erratic behavior exists at a low level of consciousness which must be surpassed to become a consistent performer.* 99

Critical Thinking Question

Have you really made a decision to succeed on your diet, or are you playing with it like a toy? If you're 100% compliant on your eating and exercise, you're serious. If you're 99% compliant, you're kidding yourself, and this is just another failed attempt to get fit.

Action Step

Adopt the belief that 99% compliance is complete failure of your diet. It's like saying you're 99% faithful in your marriage. Only accept 100% compliance from yourself.

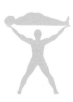

Fat people become emotionally overwhelmed with their diet

Fit people compartmentalize their emotions and methodically move from step to step

Middle-class thinkers allow their emotions to control their thoughts and dictate their behavior. Out of control, rollercoaster emotions are what lead to yo-yo dieting. That's why the masses actually believe dieting doesn't work. The truth is, their lack of emotional control is the real problem. Fit people have mastered their emotions to the point of using them to their advantage when they're positive and keeping them under control when they're not. While fat people experience emotional highs and lows, fit people keep their emotions neutralized. This allows them to perform consistently day after day, no matter what's happening around them. They build this emotional control by monitoring their thoughts, feelings and attitudes and directing them to serve their own best interests. They train themselves to avoid emotional eating of any kind, and they refuse to miss an exercise session simply because they're not in the mood. Fit people know that emotions are tricky, and giving in to them for even one meal is a slippery slope. Once their emotions are under control and helping them move forward, fit people continue to keep a close watch knowing that one emotional swing can knock them off course. They treat their emotions like a pet rattlesnake that can never be completely trusted or left alone. Some people find this habit easier to build than others, but everyone who wants world-class results has to build it, no matter how long it takes. Their secret is mentally organizing their emotions into compartments, and only allowing themselves to think about one emotion at a time. If they feel like cheating on their diet, they deal with that emotion until they redirect it. If they're too tired to exercise, they alter their emotions to generate the energy necessary to stay on track. While fat people are slaves to their emotions, fit people control and manipulate them like an orchestra leader to move them closer to their health and fitness goals.

Fat Loser Quote

66 *The foundation of mental toughness is the ability to control and manipulate your emotions to serve your own best interests. Fit people experience the same emotions as fat people, but fit people are able to redirect their emotional energy towards behaviors that keep them thin and healthy. Fat people are slaves to their emotions and fit people are masters of their emotions.* 99

Critical Thinking Question

Are you thinking of your diet as one day at a time or becoming emotionally overwhelmed by thinking how you are going to lose all this weight?

Action Step

Adopt the 'one day at a time' philosophy. If you're still feeling overwhelmed, think of it as one hour at a time. Like a computer that freezes up when it has too many software programs running, your mind will underperform when too many thoughts are straining its capacity. Make this process easy to mentally manage.

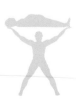

Fat people make half hearted commitments to their diet

Fit people make do or die commitments

Fat people are famous for weak commitments made in times of high emotional excitement. They're doomed to fail from the beginning because of the mindset they use. This is usually the result of seeing a photograph where they look fat or an experience where they were embarrassed by their obesity. The masses go on a diet and grit their teeth until they can't take it anymore. They fail to understand that it's their thinking that's controlling their behavior, and until they change, they will always be fat. Fit people are known for making do or die commitments and sticking to them as ferociously as a tiger. They've learned that one of critical traits of a champion is the ability to make a commitment and do whatever it takes to fulfill it. While fat people are cutting back on unhealthy foods and only exercising when they feel like it, fit people stay 100% compliant to their plan of action. More than anything else, fat people love to be comfortable. Fit people sacrifice short term comfort for long term success. They've learned that the ability to keep a commitment is a habit that separates the world class from the middle class. It goes far beyond losing and maintaining weight. Fit people make a decision and then use their willpower to stick to it no matter what obstacles they encounter. While the media and so called experts are claiming willpower doesn't work in dieting, fit people are getting healthier every day using it.

Fat Loser Quote

❝ *Getting fit is a commitment you make to yourself. No one cares if you get fit. They can barely handle their own problems. This is about you. You were born alone and you will die alone, and in between those two dates it's your job to take care of yourself. Like being born and dying, no matter how many loved ones you have at your side, getting fit is a journey you take on your own. Love and support are extremely helpful, but in the end you either keep your commitment to yourself or you don't.* ❞

Critical Thinking Question

If you were being tried in a court of law for being 100% committed to your diet and exercise plan, would there be enough evidence to convict you?

Action Step

Examine your commitment level to getting fit from your actions of the last seven days. If you're off track, forgive yourself and start over today on the path of 100% compliance.

Fat people lack the confidence to stick to their diet

Fit people have supreme self-confidence

Fat people have lied to themselves so many times about diet and exercise that they lack the confidence to adhere to any decision long term. Fit people have built world-class credibility with themselves and the confidence to manifest any vision they create. They develop this confidence by consistently keeping their word to themselves, no matter what they're doing. Their confidence gives them the belief that the only variable in the weight loss/maintenance process is the diet. Fit people know they'll stick to their diet no matter what happens, which ensures their success. The secret to building supreme self- confidence from scratch is making small commitments to yourself and keeping them. One by one, these little successes add up until you begin to believe you will finish everything you start, no matter how uncomfortable it gets. Start with 100% compliance to your diet and exercise program, even if you don't lose any weight in the short term. Your weight loss is not as important as the self-confidence you will build by sticking to your diet and exercise program. Within a few short months of 100% compliance, you will be losing weight, feeling great, and be on your way to world-class self-confidence that will have a positive impact on every aspect of your life. Resist the temptation to break your commitment, even for one meal or exercise session. Remember it's not the slight deviation in your diet or exercise that makes cheating so dangerous, it's weakening the habit you're trying to build. When you're fit and healthy and your habits are rock solid, you'll have your share of meals where you can safely deviate. But in the beginning, it's critical that you stick to the plan and build your self-confidence day by day.

Fat Loser Quote

66 *Nothing builds self-confidence like success. A fat person who sticks to her diet and exercise program will develop more confidence every day. In the beginning, her confidence will grow in linear fashion. As time goes on, her confidence will grow exponentially with each success until it reaches the level of supreme self-confidence. This non-linear growth only kicks in when she achieves one success after another, and that's why the masses rarely experience it. Once supreme self-confidence is achieved, she believes she can accomplish anything, and the upward spiral to world-class success is set in motion. Are you starting to understand why you must get fit? Your level of success, your feelings of fulfillment and your overall happiness depend on it.* 99

Fat people are unaware of their beliefs and philosophies about dieting

Fit people are hyper-aware of all of their beliefs and philosophies

Fat people believe being fit is about finding the right diet. The truth is, there are hundreds of world-class diets and they're easy to follow if you're committed. Fit people know if you want to change any behavior in your life the key is to go directly to the root of the problem, which are the beliefs and philosophies of the individual. Our beliefs dictate our behaviors, and fat people have a set of beliefs that direct them to be fat no matter how great their diet is. Here are a few distinctions in beliefs between fat and fit people: Fat people see dieting as drudgery that can only be tolerated for shorts periods of time. Fit people see dieting as a strategy for a lifetime to keep them healthy, looking good and feeling great. Fat people feel as though they're depriving themselves of their favorite foods. Fit people know they can eat their favorite foods as long as they're at their ideal weight and the deviation is well planned. Fat people believe exercise is an added burden in their life. Fit people see daily exercise as a mandatory habit for optimum physical and mental health and longevity. As you can see, fat people have been programmed to fail before they ever start a new diet. Their middle-class beliefs virtually guarantee their failure. The secret is to change your beliefs and philosophies one by one by upgrading the way you use the language with yourself and others. The next step is to become hyper-aware of all your beliefs and philosophies so you can keep the ones that serve you and upgrade the ones that don't. Start spending more time with fit people, and question them about their beliefs around diet and exercise. The most fit people are usually the most aware of their thinking in this area. Immerse your consciousness in world-class beliefs by reading books and listening to audio programs and podcasts by people who have mastered their thinking. It won't take long to understand why these people are so fit and healthy. It all begins with the way you think.

Fat Loser Quote

66 *The single best belief you can build about dieting is 'I am always 100% compliant on my diet.' The single best belief you can build about exercise is 'I exercise every day.' Remember that beliefs create behaviors, and behaviors drive results.* 99

Critical Thinking Question

Are you really aware of your fundamental beliefs and philosophies that relate to health and fitness?

Action Step

Make a list of your five most deeply held beliefs about eating and exercise. Then ask yourself if they are helping or hurting you?

Fat people make choices that keep them fat

Fit people make choices that keep them fit

All of us choose to be fat or fit. No one forces us to eat the way we eat or exercise or not. We are 100% responsible for what we see in the mirror. It all comes down to the choices we make every day during meal times and exercise periods. Fat people are famous for deluding themselves when it comes to these facts, which is the primary reason they're fat. It's not the food manufacturers' fault we get fat. It's not the fast food chains or advertisers. It's us. Fit people make conscious food choices at every meal. Fat people eat unconsciously and emotionally, ignoring the fact they're digging their own grave with a knife and fork. When they do make conscious food choices, they choose the wrong foods while promising that tomorrow will be different. Of course tomorrow never comes. They choose to fail day after day by lying to themselves. Before they know it, they're 25 pounds overweight. Then 35, and 50 and so on. After a few years of poor choices, they are obese, diabetic and a candidate for a heart attack. Their seemingly small choices piled up enough to threaten and maybe even end their life prematurely. Fit people are aware of the impact of their daily food and exercise choices and commit themselves to making selections that serve their long term best interests. They can afford to choose something off their diet once in a while because the majority of their choices are healthy. Fit people enjoy cheat meals far more than fat people because there is no guilt involved. It's a completely different experience cheating when you're a physical specimen than it is when you're a heart attack waiting to happen. Fit people set themselves up to enjoy the health, energy and confidence that accompanies being fit, and they also enjoy being able to afford eating their favorite foods from time to time without mental and emotional baggage putting a damper on the pleasure of the experience.

Fat Loser Quote

66 *You're fat or fit because of the choices you've made in eating and exercise. There is no other reason. No one held you down and stuffed doughnuts into your mouth. Start making choices like a fit person and you will get fit. That's all there is to it. It works 100% of the time for 100% of the people. The only variable in this equation is you. Are you ready to start making healthier choices? Do you really want to be fat forever? Are you ready to turn your pain and frustration into action? Then stop thinking about it and go do it!* 99

Critical Thinking Question

Are most of your choices around health and fitness more middle class or world class?

Action Step

Choose today to make only world-class choices in your eating and exercise, knowing that your ongoing choices are the foundation of your habits, and your habits will determine your results.

Fat people eat for instant pleasure

Fit people eat for delayed gratification

Fat people use food like a drug to alter the way they feel. Every few hours, the food junkie needs another fix to keep his emotions high. This eating for instant pleasure addiction is easy to develop and requires commitment and courage to break. Fit people have a vision of exactly what they want to look and feel like, and they eat according to the diet they believe will get them there. Fit people recognize the dangers of eating for instant pleasure as well as how quickly this mild sin can become a deadly habit. The key to breaking this addiction is to find other methods of altering your states of mind. Fit people use exercise to enhance the pleasure they experience. They get a double benefit in the weight loss/maintenance process. The endorphins released during exercise create feelings of happiness and well being, not to mention the natural high that occurs by knowing you're doing something that's really good for you. Many fit people get involved in sports that make exercising more fun while giving them instant pleasure. The list of activities to replace instant pleasure eating is endless. All it requires is a little creativity and the desire to change. Fat people believe changes like this require great discipline, but fit people know that building a new habit gets a little easier every day. The most painful part of the process is making the decision to do it. It's all downhill after that. That's not to say you won't have challenges along the way, but they will get easier and easier to overcome. Three to four weeks of steady progress and all that's required after that is a light discipline to maintain the habit you've constructed. Fat people scoff at the suggestion that habit change is this simple while fit people have been capitalizing on it for years. Why not follow the winners?

Fat Loser Quote

Instant pleasure is the choice of a child. Delayed gratification is the choice of a grown up. The one you choose most often indicates whether you think like an adult or more like an adolescent.

Critical Thinking Question

Are you using food as a drug to alter your emotional states of mind or do you view it as your body's primary fuel source?

Action Step

Start to monitor the reason you're eating what you're eating and when you're eating it. This will give you a glimpse of why you're getting the results you're getting.

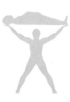

Fat people see themselves as failures

Fit people see themselves as comeback artists

Fat people are in the habit of reliving their past failures over and over, to the point where they begin to see themselves as failures. Fit people know that failing is just a result, not a judgment. All of us have failed, especially at dieting. Every fit person I know has a story of failing at some point in his or her evolution. But while fat people are wallowing in thoughts of failure, fit people see themselves as mentally tough enough to make a comeback. They believe it doesn't matter how many times you fail, but how often you succeed. They believe failure allows us to begin again more intelligently, so that's what they do. The irony of fat people who make a comeback and get fit is they seem to enjoy the victory much more than the person who succeeds the first time they try. Fit people who have failed in the past, or succeeded but gained the weight back report feelings of sustained fulfillment after their ultimate success. They know what it feels like to lose and win, and that gives them perspective from both sides. The beautiful truth is, if you've failed at dieting in the past and you're willing to get tough and change, you're more likely to experience massive success and enjoy it. There's a level of satisfaction and appreciation you can't get any other way. Another benefit of this psychological phenomenon is it applies to every other area of our lives, and the great ones know it. This is one of the reasons fit people are usually far more successful in every aspect of their lives. They've discovered one of the great secrets of world-class success: Everything affects everything.

Fat Loser Quote

❝ Most of us have been fat at some point in our lives. Big deal. Stop beating yourself up and start seeing yourself as a comeback artist. You know exactly how to get fit and you've made the decision to do it. In 30 days of 100% compliance you'll be on an emotional high you won't believe, and on your way to being thin and healthy. All your past failures are stepping stones to the new you. So get excited and go for it! ❞

Critical Thinking Question

Have you forgiven yourself for getting fat?

Action Step

Forgive yourself for all your past failures and decide to start your life over today. Everything you're not happy with is now considered a 'do over'.

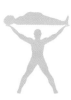

Fat people diet their way

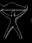

Fit people are coachable

Fat people believe the thinking that made them fat will make them thin. Fit people ask for help and are coachable. They know if successful dieting was just a matter of making a few modifications, everyone would be thin and healthy. The truth is fit people think very differently about food than fat people, and their thinking is the foundation of their success. Fat people must be re-trained in this area or they will continue to fail. The fastest way to alter your beliefs and philosophies is to get coaching from someone who can help. This is why we started the Fat Losers Program back in 2003. This 12-week telecourse is a no-nonsense mental toughness training program for weight loss and maintenance. Participants who cheat on their diet or exercise program are immediately ejected from the class. All the coaches are past graduates who have successfully maintained their weight loss. This program is not for the faint of heart or the easily offended. It's designed for people who are serious and willing to commit to their health and fitness without excuses. It will definitely show you what you're made of. The fact is, there are many good coaching programs out there to assist you in your journey. Fat people often act as lone wolves who think getting help is a sign of weakness. They let their egos get in the way of their success, and in a few short weeks they're right back where they started. Regular exposure to a world-class coach will not only motivate you, it will educate you in how a fit person thinks. They see food and exercise very differently than fat people, and just listening to them talk will show you what you need to change in your own thoughts, philosophies, and habits.

Critical Thinking Question

Are you letting your ego get in
the way of getting help?

Action Step

If you're succeeding by yourself, then stick with it.
If not, get a coach to help you get fit. Remember,
the only thing that matters is the result. Refuse
to let foolish pride interfere with your success.

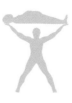

Fat people give into cravings

Fit people remain compliant

Fat people believe they can cave in to cravings without consequences. Fit people know caving in is a slippery slope that leads to obesity. Fat people treat dieting like a toy they can play with whenever they feel like it. The truth is your life is at stake, whether you know it or not. Fat people get sick from being fat. Sometimes they die from it. Dieting is not a toy, a game or a hobby. Its serious business and it must be approached as such. Cravings are like mini-addictions that must be mastered. The best thing about overcoming cravings is they become less powerful every time you conquer them. Your success is this process sends a clear message from your mind to your body that says "I'm in control and you're not. I'm the master and you're the servant. Stop craving foods you can't have." Fat people feel helpless to stop themselves while fit people are in total control. You begin by taking control over cravings and that sets the stage for the ultimate victory: taking control of your diet and exercise. . .and finally. . .your entire life. Fit people carry their success into everything they do. While fat people believe being fit is only about their health and looks, the truth is, your success in this area will make you richer, more fulfilled and happier. If you can conquer cravings, eventually, you will be able to conquer anything. Fit people use the same focus, discipline, concentration and tenacity as successful people in any area of life. The principles are the same and simple to follow. It may not be easy in the beginning, but every time you choose to ignore a craving it will get a little easier. All you have to do after that is stand guard and block the old habits from returning.

Fat Loser Quote

❝ 100% compliance is the key to your success. Bitch, moan and complain if you choose, but always stay compliant. A bad attitude won't keep you fat, but cheating on your diet will. ❞

Critical Thinking Question

Do you have a plan in place to handle cravings?

Action Step

Develop a detailed emergency plan to handle sudden cravings. Don't allow momentary desires to derail your diet due to inadequate preparation.

Fat people display their conviction with words

Fit people display their conviction with action

Fat people talk a great game. They'll spend hours justifying why they're fat and the reason dieting and exercise don't work. Fit people skip the talk and go straight to work. They prove themselves to themselves and others by their results. Being fit or fat is something you can't hide. No words are necessary. When you walk down the street the world knows whether you're winning or losing the health and fitness game. Fat people waste a lot of time explaining their failure, while fit people just keep working at success. The mental toughness message is simple: get tough and go to work. Stop philosophizing and speculating about how and why you are fat. No one cares. All your friends and loved ones care about is you getting thin and healthy. The past is gone, so get over it and move forward. You're not the first person to get fat and you won't be the last. Most of us have gained too much weight at some time in our lives. It doesn't make you any less of a human being because you wolfed down too many doughnuts and pizzas. Focus on the future and fix the problem. Stop talking about all the times you've lost weight and gained it back. Everyone has. So what. What counts is that this time you're playing to win and you're ready to fight for your health. The past is gone and your future looks brighter than ever. Follow fit people and take action. You're closer than you think to a beautiful, healthy body you can be proud of and a level of self-confidence you won't believe. All you have to do is take one step at a time.

Fat Loser Quote

" Stop talking about your diet and start taking action. Your words mean nothing unless you're doing what it takes to get fit, and you can't hide being fat. If you're taking action you will succeed. Decide to be a doer instead of a big mouth, and go out and show the world what you're made of. "

Critical Thinking Question

Do your results prove you to be a person of big talk or big action?

Action Step

Keep taking daily action in your eating and exercise habits whether you feel like it or not. Talk big or stay quiet, but remember that your actions are the only thing that counts.

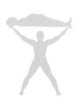

Fat people make decisions slowly and change them quickly

Fit people make decisions quickly and change them slowly

Fat people suffer from a lack of self-confidence because they believe they can't control what they eat. The truth is they can control anything they want to, if they would only make the decision to do it. As a result, fat people are cautious in decision making because they don't trust themselves. Fit people make decisions quickly because they trust their instincts. They rarely change their decisions because even when their instincts are wrong, they know they will find a way to make the decision work in their favor. They rely heavily on themselves. They believe their opinion is just as or more important than anyone else's. Some of this confidence and self-trust comes from winning the weight loss/maintenance battle. Very few people can call themselves fit. Obesity is an epidemic, and anyone who is fit and healthy stands out in the crowd as a winner. Fit people are seen as role models to be admired. They serve as a beacon of hope to the seemingly hopeless. They are seen as leaders who are strong and decisive. They are out in front showing us the way. Their decisiveness carries over into every area of their lives, both personally and professionally. And the more quality decisions they make, the more confident they get. Their success feeds on itself and makes them stronger every day. When they look in the mirror they see a well sculpted piece of human art that's been meticulously maintained. Can you imagine? Is it any wonder they have the confidence to do anything they set their mind to?

Critical Thinking Question

Are you a person that sticks to your good decisions, or do you allow your emotions to get the best of you and make commitments you can't keep?

Action Step

Practice making decisions all day today, and be consciously aware of what motivated you to make them. Once you understand your psychological habit patterns, it will be easier to catch yourself before you make mistakes.

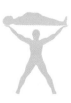

Fat people choose pleasure over discipline

Fit people choose discipline over pleasure

Fat people focus on foods that taste good, no matter what the long term cost may be. Fit people exercise discipline by putting long term results ahead of immediate pleasure. It's not that fit people are more disciplined than fat people, they simply engage their discipline when they eat and exercise. There are many world-class performers in other areas of life who are extremely disciplined in their area of focus, yet fail to transfer that discipline to their dietary habits. The sad thing is many of these people choose to exercise their discipline in business while ignoring their health and this grave error in judgment costs some of them their lives. It's hard to enjoy the fruits of your labor if you're dead. Fit people are acutely aware of this and choose to gain their pleasure from the increased energy, vitality and overall good health they experience as a result of developing disciplined dietary/exercise habits. Both the fat and the fit gain pleasure from eating, but while one is short term and potentially deadly, the other offers almost unlimited physical and psychological benefits. Fit people get the added benefit of looking and feeling successful as a byproduct of their discipline and mental toughness. They stand out among the crowd, most of whom are either a little fat, very fat, or obese. Fit people are looked up to as role models and winners in a game most people are losing. They have an advantage in business, relationships, and many other areas of life simply because they're fit. We're all taught not to judge a book by its cover, and it's a nice philosophy we should all follow. But we all know that's not how the world works. People judge people by the way they look, right or wrong. Why not give yourself every advantage you can get?

Fat Loser Quote

❝ Discipline is an investment and pleasure is an expenditure. Invest in your fitness every day by staying 100% compliant, and you will reap the pleasure of abundant health for the rest of your life. Fat people allow their mental energy to focus on the pleasure of eating and cheating, while fit people are strategically directing their thoughts to the wonderful future that awaits them when all of their disciplined investments pay off. ❞

Critical Thinking Question

Are you aware of the danger of consistently choosing pleasure over discipline?

Action Step

Begin to monitor whether you're choosing pleasure over discipline or discipline over pleasure in all areas of your life. Look for correlations between your successes and the times you choose discipline.

Fat people refuse to let go of the foods that made them fat

Fit people do whatever it takes to stay fit

Fat people are more concerned about being able to gorge on foods they think bring them instant happiness than they are about getting thin and healthy. They believe sacrificing unhealthy foods that will eventually lead them into type two diabetes, high cholesterol and a host of other debilitating diseases is too high of a price to pay for optimum health, boundless energy and renewed enthusiasm for life. Fat people focus their determination on not having to change. Fit people focus their determination on doing whatever it takes to serve their own best interests. They make a decision to get thin and healthy and stick to it until they accomplish their goal. While fat people fight to hold on to their old habits and sink deeper and deeper into failing health, fit people let go of their old habits and climb higher and higher every day into world-class fitness. The irony is that both groups possess a fierce determination to get what they want, and they usually both succeed. Fat people are the architects of their own destruction. All they have to do is direct the same determination it took to hold on to their old eating/exercise habits and point it toward a more positive approach. Both groups have the same amount of mental power. It's how they choose to use it that makes the difference between thriving health and early death. If you're fat and stuck in this rut, the secret is taking the first small step: decide to do whatever it takes to get thin and healthy. This problem can't be ignored and it's only going to get worse. Kill the monster while it's little.

Make a decision and go for it! People with far less determination and focus have gone from fat to fit, and you can, too. Why not start today?

Fat Loser Quote

" *Adopt the ultimate goal achieving, dream manifestation mindset of world-class performers: 'whatever it takes'. Decide you will bear any burden and endure any hardship to get fit and your whole life will change. This is how the great ones go from success to success. They're not any smarter than us, but their resolve is as solid as steel. Decide to adopt this philosophy today.* "

Critical Thinking Question

What price are you willing to pay to get fit?
Are you really willing to do whatever it takes?

Action Step

Identify your current level of commitment in the weight loss process. On a scale of 1-7, 7 being 'whatever it takes' and 1 being no commitment at all, how do you rank? Anything but a 7 means you're headed for failure.

Fat people expect
to lose and gain weight forever

Fit people expect
to build the body of their dreams

F at people buy into the mass belief that dieting is an up and down process by nature. Fit people know this is not necessary, nor is it a good
strategy. Breaking any habit takes between 21-30 days of 100% compliance with your diet and fitness programs, and after that it's simply a matter of guarding the door anytime the old habits come calling. The first 30
days require discipline and commitment. After that, it only requires a light
discipline to maintain your fitness. This is why fit people fully expect from
the beginning to build the body of their dreams. They cut out pictures
of people they want to look like at their ideal weight and inundate their
consciousness with these images every day. As their weight drops, their
excitement grows and their belief increases. Every day they move closer
to the picture and their momentum becomes a force to reckon with. They
begin to imagine what they will feel like at their perfect weight, and how
their life will be better as a result. They visualize the compliments they
will get from others and the built-in advantages they will have as a fit
person in a world full of fat people. Every meal and workout makes them
physically and psychologically stronger until they begin to believe they
can accomplish anything. It affects their attitude and outlook on life to the
point that it starts to impact the people around them. There's nothing as
infectious as a winner on the road to another victory! Their energy is pal-
pable, and it feels great just being in their presence. So while fat people are

expecting to ride the failure-success-failure rollercoaster, this middle-class self-fulfilling prophecy never enters the minds of the great ones. They expect to win and they do. Over and over. They are no different than you and I, except in their thinking.

Fat Loser Quote

66 *Expectations rule the world. Human beings get exactly what they expect. Unfortunately, most people don't expect much and the universe is happy to fulfill that expectation. Fat people expect to be fatter tomorrow than they are today, and that's what they get. Fit people expect to be in better shape at 50 than they were at 20, and the universe is happy to fulfill that wish as well. So if the universe is happy to fulfill any expectation you have, why not expect the best? Your world-class expectation combined with a solid work ethic will manifest results most people wouldn't believe were even possible.* 99

Critical Thinking Question

Are your expectations more
middle class or world class?

Action Step

Expectations are self-imposed and can be
upgraded at any time. Decide today to expect
to develop the body of your dreams. Look for
pictures in magazines of people with bodies
you would like to have and tape them on
poster board so you can see them every day.
Build this image in your mind and expect it
to happen. This will drive you to behave in
ways that lead you to your expected result.

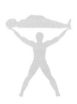

Fat people are enthusiastic about their diet until they get hungry

Fit people are enthusiastic about being hungry

Fit people know being hungry for short periods of time is the opportunity to drop excess weight. So they actually condition themselves to respond enthusiastically to hunger. It's not that they enjoy feeling hungry, but they learn to become enthusiastic about it because they are focused on their long term weight loss goal. Fat people are forever searching for the pain free way to weight loss success, and it doesn't exist. Successful people in any area of life all know every success comes with a non-negotiable price tag. Doctors, chemists, and other dietary formulators have made the weight loss process simpler than ever, but not easy. You will pay a price for fitness. The reality is that if you choose not to pay it, you'll pay an even higher price for being fat. Critical thinking in this arena is pretty clear: the only intelligent choice is to get thin and healthy. . .now, while you still have a choice! The clock is ticking. Why not make up your mind while you're still in control? If you don't act first, disease will act for you. There's only one reasonable choice to make. This is why fit people are able to maintain their world-class enthusiasm when the rest of us are complaining about not being able to pig out on pizzas, beer and chips. If you think training yourself to be enthusiastic when you're hungry is simply a positive thinking platitude, think again. Remember Dr. Pavlov and his dogs. Classical conditioning is science that can be used by anyone. It just depends on how badly you want to win the battle of the bulge. If failing only leads to disease, embarrassment, and a mediocre existence, is it really even an option? Why not direct the power of your enthusiasm toward winning this war and maximizing your potential? Don't you deserve to be happy and healthy? Of course you do! So get started today.

Fat Loser Quote

66 *Become acutely aware of your internal focus. If you're focused on your next meal, short term hunger pangs are painful. If you're focused on losing weight, short term hunger pangs mean progress. The event is the same, but your internal focus will determine its meaning to you.* **99**

Critical Thinking Question

What does being hungry on your diet mean to you? Could you reframe this meaning to better serve your best interests?

Action Step

Identify all the so called negative parts of dieting and exercising and start to redefine them one by one. To the masses, being sore after a workout is negative. To the great ones, being sore is a sign of progress. One definition leads to motivation, and the other to negative thoughts that lead to failure. It's your mind. Define everything in a way that serves you.

Fat people love to eat more than they love feeling fit

Fit people love feeling fit more than they love to eat

S ome things in life are unparalleled. The feeling of being in love. The feeling of winning. The feeling of making a difference in someone else's life. These are a few of life's unique and special gifts. The joy of being lean, healthy and fit is another that is in a class by itself. The feeling you get looking in the mirror every morning and being proud of what you see cannot be purchased with any amount of money. That's one of the reasons it feels so good: it must be earned through discipline, sacrifice and mental toughness, and everyone knows it. Fit people are treated better than fat people. I'm not saying it's right, only stating a fact. Fit people are definitely favored and respected more than fat people in society. Again, this is just the way the world works. Instead of fighting or denying it, fit people see it for what it is and develop a strategy to win the game. They are willing to fight and win this battle because the feeling of being fit and all its associated benefits are worth far more than having unlimited access to cheeseburgers, French fries and doughnuts. Fat people have either never experienced the magical feeling of fitness, or they have forgotten it. If they recalled this, they'd never have let themselves get out of shape. It wouldn't even be a close decision. Loving to eat is an addiction that can be broken. Loving the feeling of world-class fitness is the path to health and happiness. Fit people learn to love the foods that keep them thin and healthy, while occasionally enjoying anything they feel like eating. Being fit doesn't mean giving up hot fudge sundaes forever, it means being strategic as to when you eat them and how much you eat. It's the difference between drinking yourself into a drunken stupor and having a few beers when your strategy says you can afford the calories. One approach is what the masses often practice, and the other is how world-class thinkers approach everything they do: consciously. Conscious eating; conscious fitness.

Fat Loser Quote

Fitness is the physical equivalent of being wealthy. It's a feeling of total abundance, as if you're living in a world where you make the rules and anything is possible. Obstacles that were once insurmountable are easily conquered. It's a feeling of personal control and self-mastery. You wake up every day basking in the glow of self-respect and supreme confidence, ready to accept any challenge you're confronted with because you're a winner. You beat the odds. You know it, and everyone around you knows it.

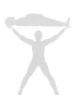

Fat people associate with fat people

Fit people associate with fit people

There's a piece of ancient wisdom all of us have heard: you'll become just like the people with whom you spend the most time. If you're an alcoholic, chances are you hang out in bars or with other people who drink too much. If you're broke, odds are your closest friends have money problems. And if you're fat, you probably have fat friends and family in your inner circle. Fit people usually hang out with other fit people, and together, they strengthen each other's discipline, resolve, and mental toughness. This means if you're fat, it's time to make some new friends! That doesn't mean you have to drop your fat friends, but seriously limiting the time you spend with them is sage advice. It's not an elitist move, but a practical one. Consciousness is contagious and what you catch can help or hurt you. Your job is to start spending time with people who value their health and fitness more than their gluttonous desires. Start by joining a health club. Get to know some of the members there who are diligently, every day, sweating their way to better health and longer life. Fit people see the world differently than fat people, and you must become intimately acquainted with their deepest core beliefs and philosophies. Exposure to their work ethic will impress, inspire and motivate you to greater action. After a short while, you will begin seeing the world though their eyes as you get thinner and healthier. Feed off their belief and enthusiasm until you're strong enough to feed off your own. That's the upside. The downside is some of your fat friends may take offense at your new way of thinking and may even be envious of your success. Anyone who has broken away from the masses has experienced this. Let me be the first to empathize with you, and at the same time rejoice in your new success. Part of the price of winning is the jealousy and envy of the mediocre, middle-class mindset. Don't let it get you down, because you're in good company. The wealthiest people in the world pay the most in taxes and give the most money away, yet are scorned by the masses. Couples with great relationships are looked at with skepticism by the middle class. And fit people are called everything from self-centered to shallow to narcissistic. Being a winner has a price, but the price of losing is deadly. Make a list of all your closest friends and write down whether they are fit or fat, and then make a commitment to add five new fit people to your inner circle. The exposure alone will be worth the effort.

Fat Loser Quote

66 *If you want to be rich, hang around rich people. If you want to be happy, hang around happy people. And if you want to be fit, hang around fit people. Fat people are every bit as good as fit people, except in their thinking in the area of diet and exercise. Fit people know how to think about diet and exercise and that's why they're fit. The more time you invest in positioning yourself in the presence of success, the more successful you will become. If this strategy offends you, get over it, because it's too important to miss. Did you really think you were going to get fit by thinking the same way you've always thought? Push yourself to expand your thinking and new opportunities beyond your wildest dreams will begin to present themselves.* 99

Critical Thinking Question

In your inner circle of closest friends, how many of them are fat and how many are fit?

Action Step

Begin building relationships with fit people who will have a positive impact on your thinking. Cut back on time spent with those who haven't mastered this area of their life until you're strong enough to be unaffected by them.

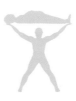

Fat people never have enough time to exercise

Fit people always find enough time to exercise

The primary difference between fit and fat people is in their thinking around the critical habits of optimum health, none of which is more important than exercise. Fat people see exercise as something that only gets done after every other priority during their day has been completed. They fail to recognize that exercise is not a hobby, but a way of life to maintain good health. To fit people, exercise is a religion and law. It's one of their top priorities during the day, and if they happen to miss even a single workout, they feel sloppy, slothful and guilty. It's a healthy addiction. A fit person will do almost anything to maintain the physical and psychological momentum their exercise routine offers. Visit any health club between 6 and 9pm and you'll see the same dedicated group lifting weights, running on the treadmill and participating in exercise classes. Contrary to the criticism leveled at these people by the middle class, gym rats are one of the most disciplined sub-cultures in society. They show up day after day, or night after night, and while the masses are surfing the Internet, playing video games and eating pizza, they're building bodies that generate energy, enthusiasm and self-esteem. For most fit people, it's not about developing huge muscles or rock hard abs, it's about fostering excellent health, maintaining their ideal weight and looking and feeling great. Fit people exercise at home, on the road and anywhere they have to, no matter what it takes. While fat people require perfect conditions to exercise, fit people know the only perfect condition is a mindset rooted in commitment. They set exercise goals, read exercise magazines, and socialize with other fit people. It's a large part of their daily consciousness. The first step to make exercise a priority is your decision to include it in your daily schedule and stick to it. In four weeks you'll wonder how you ever lived without it.

Fat Loser Quote

66 *World-class fitness demands you make daily exercise one of the highest priorities in your life. It's no longer something you do when you have time. It must become as routine as brushing your teeth and taking a shower, to the point where you don't feel right if you miss it. This habit is critical to your success. It's one of the most important habits you'll ever build, and the payoff is enormous.* 99

Critical Thinking Question

Are you placing enough priority on your exercise time, or is it the first thing that gets eliminated during a busy day?

Action Step

Decide today to make exercise one of your top priorities, and build the habit of working out every day.

Fat people put faith in their diet

Fit people put faith in themselves

F at people expect their diet to make them fit. They put all their faith in their diet, and when the going gets tough they blame their diet for failing. This is why the middle class coined the phrase, "diets don't work", which will go down in human history as the grandest health delusion of all time. Diets don't fail people; people fail diets. . .and then blame the diet! It's like not showing up for class and saying school doesn't work. It's a ridiculous statement that's become such a major part of the American lexicon that many people actually believe it. Even though diets work, fit people put their faith where it belongs: in themselves. They trust themselves to pick the right diet and exercise program, and more importantly, they trust themselves to follow it until they succeed. They carry this faith into everything they do, and it's the foundation of their success. When they achieve their ideal weight, they know they will be able to maintain it. While the masses rely on outside forces, world-class thinkers are self-reliant and strong. They have the street smarts to understand no one can make them fit and healthy but themselves. They are grounded in objective reality which tells them being fit is the natural order of human existence. People are supposed to be lean and healthy, not fat and sick. Restaurants might serve oversized portions, food manufacturers might use too many addictive ingredients, and advertisers might be guilty of promoting unhealthy choices; but in the final analysis, each of us is 100% responsible for being fat or fit. That's objective reality, and no amount of spin or delusional thinking can change it. Everyone who wishes to evolve from fat to fit must eventually realize they are the secret to their own success. The masses will always live in a victim mentality. The middle-class mindset thrives on feeling sorry for itself. It's a form of pleasure that allows failure without accepting responsibility. Fit people break through this self-destructive conditioning and join the ranks of champions. Then they apply their world-class thinking to anything they focus on, and fitness is usually near the top of the list, because it impacts everything they do. The secret to joining the fit begins by believing in yourself, even if you never have before. Make no mistake: you can do it.

Fat Loser Quote

❝ Above all else, you have to believe in yourself. You have to let go of the fear of failing on your diet, no matter how many times you've failed, and trust yourself to do whatever it takes. No one can do this for you. People can support you, love you, and cheer you on from the sidelines, but in the end, it all comes down to you. This kind of faith requires that you forgive yourself for all past failures and make a fresh start today. Build faith in yourself one day at a time, or even one meal at a time. Slowly, steadily, surely, your confidence will grow until it's stronger than oak. When that happens, everything else you want in your life will seem attainable. The new you is waiting for you to arrive! Don't keep her waiting! ❞

Critical Thinking Question

Are you willing to forgive yourself for the
failures of the past, and have faith enough
to believe this time will be different?

Action Step

Make a decision to take your diet and exercise
program one day at a time. You will get stronger
with each successful day and this will become
the foundation of your ultimate success.

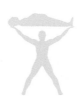

Fat people focus on their present weight

Fit people focus on their future weight

Fat people wallow in the present day problem, which keeps them from tapping into their emotional motivation. Fit people are grounded in the present, but focused on the future. They hold a mental image of themselves at their ideal weight and move toward the image. This strategy keeps them excited, motivated and inspired. As they move closer and closer to their goal, their belief gets stronger and their excitement grows. The mental image of their perfect body becomes so clear over time, they actually get to experience the feeling that will accompany their success. This makes them even stronger and more determined to make the image a reality. Fat people make the mistake of looking at their current weight and thinking about how far they have to go and how much sacrifice and suffering they have yet to endure. They grieve over the loss of being able to eat their favorite foods whenever they want. After a short period of this non-constructive thinking, most fat people give in to their own limited thinking and go off their diet. They usually don't quit the diet; they simply don't stay 100% compliant. That way they can justify their behavior to themselves. Quitting outright would be total failure, but 99% compliance to a fat person is easy to mentally resolve. They think to themselves, "Look how much I've improved my eating. I might not be 100%, but I'm better than I was." Fit people know a philosophy like that is a blueprint for failure. This is the thinking that makes people fat in the first place. Successful dieting is all or nothing.

Make a decision, stick to it and lose weight or prepare yourself for the fact that you are going to die fat. The masses think they can beat the system by thinking fat and getting fit. Why torture yourself believing you're going to be thin and healthy if you're going to keep thinking and behaving like a fat person? Getting fit is not a hobby, it's a commitment. Either make a decision to do it, or settle for obesity. It doesn't make you any less of a person, it just makes you fat. Let it go and follow the new wave of fat people who call themselves full figured and plus-sized, and claim to be happy with it. God bless you if you can get yourself to believe that colossal lie. But if you decide to go for fitness, stop looking at where you are, and focus on where you're going. Before you know it, your vision will become reality.

Fat Loser Quote

66 *The masses focus their mental energy on the past and present, always struggling to survive. The great ones pay attention to the present, but dream of the beautiful future that currently only exists on the movie screen of their minds. While fat people are drowning in fear, self-loathing and regret, fit people are basking in the vision of their ideal future, always seeing themselves getting exactly what they want. Every day they take action that moves them closer to their perfect life. They were not born knowing how to do this. This is a learned skill. The secret is manifesting one major success in your life that sets off an atomic bomb in your brain which explodes and forces you to question every limiting belief you ever had. The more you succeed, the more you dream of the future. It's exciting to consider the possibilities when you believe you can make them come true. Your first major success should be fitness. After that, your future is limitless.* 99

Critical Thinking Question

Have you imagined what you will look
like at your ideal weight? Have you
thought about how good it will feel?

Action Step

Take thirty seconds every day
to visualize yourself living your life
as a fit and healthy person.

Fat people are incongruent

Fit people are congruent

Congruency between words and actions has always been a hallmark of the world class. When the great ones make a promise, you can take it to the bank. Among the middle class, not so much. The masses talk a good game but rarely deliver. In business, incongruence will cost you money. In health, it can cost you your life. How many fat people do you know who swear they are going to lose weight and start exercising? These promises are made so often by the average person that no one listens to them anymore, and this is where psychological incongruence destroys confidence and self-esteem. The more often you say you're going to do something and fail to do it, the less credibility you have with yourself and others. Fit people know this, and that's why they're committed to 100% meal and exercise compliance. Failing to be congruent in your diet and exercise program is not only dangerous to your health, it's a threat to your sense of well being and happiness. The downward spiral that occurs when you lie to yourself can be devastating mentally, emotionally and spiritually. It's hard to get excited about goals and dreams when you no longer trust yourself. Fit people are aware of what's at stake every time they're tempted to stray off their diet or skip a workout. So how about you? Are your habits, actions and behaviors congruent with the size and scope of your vision? If not, start over today by making a commitment to congruency. Don't get down on yourself. Every human being in the world has fallen into this trap. Make a decision right now that it won't happen again, and you'll be on your way to a body you can be proud of. Remember, no matter how fat you are right now, you can do it! All you have to do is decide to do whatever it takes.

Fat Loser Quote

❝ Always do what you say you're going to do. If you say you're going to stay 100% compliant on your diet, then do it. No excuses. No exceptions. Get tough with yourself and you can write your own ticket. If your words and actions remain incongruent, you are relegated to the lowly rewards and mediocre successes of the middle class. Do you really want to settle for second best if you don't have to? ❞

Critical Thinking Question

Do you believe you can be incongruent in your promises and actions
around weight loss and still get fit?

Action Step

Stop deluding yourself and get serious about
your health and well being. Play time is over.
It's time to grow up, get tough, and give yourself
the gift of fitness. Stop screwing around and
get on with it! The clock is ticking. Go back
to the beginning of this book and just read a
page a day to keep you on track. You really do
deserve to be fit. I believe in you. You can do it!

Fat people accept whatever they're told about dieting and exercise

Fit people only listen to other fit people

The masses believe what society tells them, no matter how much it goes against what they know to be true. Most middle-class thinkers are smart and educated, yet they allow themselves to be led down the road of mediocrity and limitation. Fit people are leaders, and often find themselves challenging the status quo and breaking through barriers the middle-class thought were impossible. Fit people know not to listen when the masses blame everything but themselves for getting fat. They know it's their fault, and they freely admit it. They know "big isn't beautiful" and not to accept being fat as their fate. When they see the media interviewing fat people claiming to be happy in their obesity, they know this is self-delusion. When they hear fat people saying they don't care that they're fat, diabetic and disease prone, they're not gullible enough to actually believe it. Fit people are fit thinkers who think for themselves. They don't need to be told what to believe or how to live. They're smart enough to be open to education, mentoring and coaching from other fit people, but they make their own de-cisions in the end. They don't choose short term fad diets because they're popular; they do their own research and consult their fit physician to de-termine the diet that suits them best. When friends and family are not sup-portive and beg them to abandon their diet, fit people ignore them and stay 100% compliant. The path to thinking for yourself is paved with self-trust. If you've fallen into the trap of following the herd, don't feel bad, because you're in the majority. Decide today to begin challenging the thinking and behavior of the masses and watch what happens to your results.

Fat Loser Quote

66 Make no mistake: you've been being sold a false bill of goods since you were born, by people of authority, for the purpose of controlling your behavior. The government legislates morality, the schools dictate your education, and your family and the church tell you right from wrong. Fitness is no different. Psychologists tell you not to expect much so you won't be disappointed, and to accept your body the way it is. Clothing companies design giant clothes for fat people and sell them through television ads that brainwash you to believe you are beautiful the way you are. It's all about control and manipulation, and it's worked for thousands of years. Wake up and take control of your own thoughts and beliefs! Start listening to fit people and build their beliefs into your consciousness. Stop allowing the so-called experts to dictate how you should think and feel and start following people who are succeeding. 99

Critical Thinking Question

Are you taking dieting and exercise advice from fat people or fit people?

Action Step

Stop listening to fat people on how to get fit. Only take advice from people with a track record of success.

Fat people see dieting as drudgery

Fit people see dieting as fun

Since fat people see dieting as a short term solution, they rarely enjoy the process. Fit people know a world-class diet is a lifestyle you can stick to and succeed with forever, and the excitement generated from improving their looks, energy and overall health makes the process enjoyable and fun. Much like starting a new exercise program, changing your diet can be a painful in the beginning, but the promise of a better future and the bevy of benefits it brings turns pain into pleasure in a short period of time. One of the most important elements of happiness that's been passed down through the ages is always having something to look forward to. This is one of the key reasons fit people enjoy losing weight. Every day promises new results— in the mirror— and they are visible to the world. Every day brings new compliments on how they look and their new found success. Additional benefits to look forward to include increased stamina, greater vitality and an elevated feeling of optimism and sense of well being. It's a win-win-win scenario with no downside other than learning a little discipline in the beginning. Unfortunately, fat people only see the struggle and suffering they imagine they will have to endure in a short term fix to a long term problem. One group of people looks forward to a brighter future while the other only sees the battle. Same scenario, completely different ways of thinking. Is it any wonder fit people succeed and fat people fail? Why not decide today to see your diet as a long term, life changing solution that can actually be fun? Not the kind of fun you have going to an amusement park or seeing a good movie, but the kind of fun that you can only get from setting a goal and achieving it. The fun that comes from beating the odds. The fun of being fit and full of life. That fun feeling of accomplishment. The kind of fun that makes you a role model to others struggling to succeed. Why not go for it? What do you have to lose?

Fat Loser Quote

66 *Winning is fun. Getting exactly what you want is fun. Actualizing your full potential is fun. Being fat sucks. Looking fat sucks. Feeling fat is the worst of all. Dieting isn't drudgery. Drudgery is living your life with a fat, disgusting, bloated body that irritates and aggravates you every time you gaze into the mirror or see yourself in a photo. Fat people choose this drudgery because it doesn't require discipline and it happens slowly over time. It's like boiling a bullfrog. He'll jump in the water because it's warm and feels good, (like eating junk food) and before he knows it, he's cooked. Self-discipline is a small price to pay for the pride, confidence and self-respect you're going to experience as a fit person.* 99

Critical Thinking Question

Are you more focused on the means to get fit or the end result? Is a life of great health, abundant energy and superior fitness drudgery or fun?

Action Step

Start focusing your mental energy on your future as a fit and healthy person. The masses will always seek shelter from short term pain, while the great ones know they can endure anything for 21-30 days if the payoff is sufficient.

Fat people hang on to dieting failures of the past

Fit people forgive themselves for past failures and focus on the future

The masses have always been obsessed with the past, especially with failures. One of the hallmarks of middle-class thinking is using past mistakes as an excuse to back off from taking further risks. In professional sports they call this "playing not to lose". This is where you must rely on luck, fate, or your opponents break down in order to succeed. Fat people are famous for employing this strategy in the weight loss process. They will consume every magic pill and potion that's sold, and go on every fad diet they can find in order to avoid full engagement in the weight loss process. This is the thinking that made them fat, and it virtually guarantees their failure until they transcend it. Fit people keep the past where it belongs. They consciously choose to look forward, and believe that the failures of the past have no impact on the future unless we give them that power, which they refuse to do unless it serves their best interests. World-class thinking recognizes the healing power of forgiving ourselves for past failures as well as allowing ourselves to succeed in the future. When you forgive yourself, you release all of the mental energy it requires to hold on to your anger, frustration and disappointment. Now all that energy is freed up to use in helping you stay tough and succeed. Fit people harness this vast reserve of mental energy and direct it toward their weight loss goal.

So while the masses only have so many mental energy units to devote toward their future, world-class thinkers have all of their energy at their disposal. This is like having an entire army focused on a single objective. Failure is nearly impossible. Decide today to let go of the failures of the past. Even the greatest performers have failed, so love yourself enough to release yourself from the bondage of guilt and regret. This is a road every great thinker must travel, and it starts with a single decision to just let go and forgive.

Fat Loser Quote

66 *The past is gone. This diet is the only one that counts, and it's going to change your life. Not just your physical life, but your entire life because of its impact on your belief system. Do you know anyone who hasn't failed on a diet? Everyone has. Let it go and move on. You have the opportunity to essentially erase (or at least make irrelevant) every dieting failure you've had by succeeding on this one. This is your chance to rewrite your own personal history. It all begins with forgiving yourself and believing this time will be different. You're older, wiser, and more committed than ever before. This is your time to shine!* 99

Critical Thinking Question

Are you still thinking about the times you
failed to get fit in the past? Do you think
you're the only one who ever failed at this?

Action Step

Decide today to let go of the past and forgive
yourself for failing. The past does not equal
the future, and your prior failure is only going
to make your success that much sweeter.

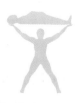

Fat people aren't sure why they're dieting

Fit people know exactly why they're dieting

Middle-class thinking allows people to get fat, and the cornerstone of middle-class thinking is delusion and denial. Fat people ignore the dangerous consequences of obesity. Even an extra 10 pounds puts enormous stress on the body that leads to disease and breakdown, not to mention depleted energy levels. Study after study shows fat to be one of our greatest enemies, yet viewed through the eyes of denial and delusion, this truth is seen as nothing more than a nuisance. That's how America can have such a high obesity rate without alarms sounding in the streets. Fit people are world-class thinkers grounded in the objective reality that there is nothing good about being fat. Critical thinking tells us it's ugly, dangerous, and life-threatening. It will hold you back from getting ahead in business, cost you relationships, and kill your sex life. Fat makes you tired, cranky and lifeless. Like it or not, those are the facts. Fit people know this and that's why they fight to change. They think of these things every time they reach for a doughnut or cheeseburger, and it keeps them on track toward their goal. When you ask a fat person why she's dieting, she'll tell you of her ongoing battle of the bulge and lament about how tough dieting is and how she struggles to find the time to exercise. The truth is she doesn't know why she's dieting, because she's been doing it for so long it's become a way of life. She will lose and gain and lose again, because she refuses to make a real commitment to solve the problem once and for all. It's not that she's undisciplined; it's that she is unclear of why she should commit. Delusion and denial have clouded her thinking. Like a junkie shooting narcotics through a needle, her thought processes in this area are hazy at best. Decide to shun delusion and live in objective reality. You are literally fighting for your life, and time is running out. Are you ready to fight?

Fat Loser Quote

❝ *Can you see yourself walking down the beach looking like a million bucks? Can you imagine what it feels like to be showered with compliments and praise from people every day because you look so good? Can you even fathom the confidence you're going to have as a result of your fitness success? Diets are scientific and logical, people are not. Identify what is driving you emotionally to get fit, and simulate those feelings in your mind every day until they're reality. This is what the masses miss. It's not about the how, it's about the why. Make sure you know what you want to feel when you arrive at your fitness goal.* ❞

Critical Thinking Question

Do you know your emotional motivators for getting fit?

Action Step

Every day, write down the five most important reasons you must get fit, until you hit your ideal weight. This will burn them into your mind and keep you on track.

Fat people believe 99% compliance is good

Fit people believe 99% compliance is terrible

The enemy of great is good. The A student is disgusted when she gets a B. The track star who misses his time by a tenth of a second considers it a failure. A fit person who has any excess fat remains unsatisfied. Most people think 99% compliance spells success. Throughout the ages, the masses have never understood that the last 1% of the equation is where victory lies! It's the difference between a world-class existence and a life of mediocrity. It's the final push to greatness that allows people to join the ranks of the great ones and write their own ticket. This ancient wisdom applies in weight loss and fitness as well. All the glory is in that last 1% of compliance. The difference between 99% and 100% compliance is like the difference between an amateur and a pro. To the masses, it's only an extra serving or a taste of dessert. To a world-class thinker, it's the destruction of a habit, and the beginning or continuation of a habitual way of thinking that says; "I can go almost all the way and succeed." Or, "I can cheat a little bit and succeed." Fat people take this into everything they do, which is why most don't get what they want. This baffles the middle-class mindset that says; 'something this simple can't be that important'. The masses are looking for the secret to success while it's right in front of them. Fit people know the power of a fully committed, made up mind. They know doing 99% of what takes to succeed is a recipe for heartache and failure. 100% is the only number that makes sense to them, and unlike the middle class, they carry this 100% philosophy into everything they do. That's why they achieve goal after goal. Society lavishes these people with praise and riches because they are so rare. But the truth is, becoming one of them is possible for any of us. One of the first steps is making a decision to go 100%. Are you ready to make that commitment to your weight loss goal?

Fat Loser Quote

❝ *If you were 99% faithful to your spouse, would that be enough for him/her? Getting fit requires 100% compliance, at least in the beginning. Once you hit your desired weight, 99% compliance may be enough to maintain it. But in the weight loss process, don't delude yourself into believing you can cheat your way through. This is the same thinking that made you fat in the first place. Break all the other rules if you wish, but stay 100% compliant and you will lose weight.* ❞

Critical Thinking Question

Are you deluding yourself into believing 99% compliance is good because it's better than what you used to do?

Action Step

Ground yourself into objective reality by waking up to the fact that getting fit is an 'all or nothing' proposition. Get serious and succeed, or quit and stay fat. The choice is yours, but treating your diet like a toy you can play with whenever you feel like it and succeed is an exercise in self-delusion.

Fat people are obsessed with food

Fit people are obsessed with success

Food is the drug of the masses. They use it to celebrate, grieve, socialize, network, boost their spirits and heal emotional wounds. The problem with the food junkie is he gets hungry every two to four hours, and the emotional high only lasts minutes. The heroin addict is high for several hours before needing the next fix. Food obsessed people need to keep feeding the monkey to remain satisfied, while at the same time having to cope with the disgust and depression of continuous weight gain. Are you starting to see why you must get tough? This isn't an eating and exercise game, it's a head game. Fit people want to succeed more than they want to eat unhealthy, fattening foods. While fat people are dreaming of pizza and beer, fit people are dreaming about walking down the street looking like a million bucks. They're ultimate success is more important than satisfying their gluttonous desires. They know gluttony lasts for minutes while success lasts for a lifetime. So while fat people are obsessing about food, fit people are seeing themselves at their ideal weight and basking in the future glory of their achievement. All this requires is a change in focus. To get started, get some poster board and paste pictures of what your ideal body will look like when you hit your goal weight. Then look at these pictures every day and you'll begin experiencing how you will feel when you look like the pictures. You'll be overwhelmed with feelings of success, fulfillment and gratitude as you move closer to your vision every day. Eating will remain an enjoyable activity but far from the focus of your life. You'll be able to eat without guilt while moving closer to your ideal weight.

Fat Loser Quote

Critical Thinking Question

Do you spend more time thinking
about eating or succeeding?

Action Step

Get past middle-class thinking by directing your
mental energy toward success. Refuse to allow
thoughts of self-pity to weaken your resolve.

Fat people think habits are something to break

Fit people know habits are something to develop

Beginning in childhood, middle-class thinking has trained people to think of habits as negative. World-class thinking associates habits with health, wealth, and success in every area of life. Good eating and exercise habits are largely ignored by the masses, and this has helped create the fattest society in the history of civilization. Fit people are acutely aware of their dominant habits because they know habitual behavior determines results. Before healthy habits are in place, the individual must be consciously aware of every thought she thinks and every move she makes. Once the proper habits are formed, behavior goes on auto-pilot like a 747 jetting through the sky. Conscious thought is no longer necessary unless the habit is in danger of being broken or compromised. Fit people build healthy habits and then stand guard to be sure they're maintained. Even the slightest deviation of a regular system or routine can begin to unravel the most established habits. This is why fit people seem borderline obsessed about what they eat. It's not the little extra food that's off their diet, but the danger of weakening a habit they worked so hard to establish. The most important habit is 100% compliance on your diet. Exercise is critical to your success, but sticking to your diet is the heart of what fit people do best. Don't cut yourself any slack in this area. 99% compliance is failing. It leads to weak habit development, substandard discipline, and it limits your confidence when you need to build it. Middle-class thinkers always seem to turn in a half-hearted effort. That's their approach to life, and that's why so many of them live lives of quiet desperation. Don't be like them! Use world-class thinking and watch your body (and your mind) transform in front of your eyes.

Fat Loser Quote

66 *Remember that it won't always be this hard. As your new habits gradually replace the old, it will get easier and easier to stick to your diet. New habits start out as cobwebs and turn into cables. Today is the toughest it will ever be.* 99

Critical Thinking Question

Do you really understand the power of being able to develop new habits at will?

Action Step

What three habits could you develop in the next 21-30 days that would have the biggest impact on your fitness?

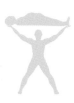

Fat people seek happiness through eating

Fit people seek happiness through achievement

A hallmark of middle-class thinking is the belief that happiness is achieved through pleasure. Fat people spend an inordinate amount of time thinking about and planning what and when they will eat. Through years of conditioning, they've learned to associate eating with their level of happiness. Fit people experience long term, lasting happiness by progressively moving toward their ideal weight and thriving on the emotional satisfaction that accompanies any act of discipline. As they get thinner and healthier, their self- confidence and momentum grows to the point where they begin to believe they can do anything. They experience feelings of gratitude for their success, which leads directly to increased happiness and life satisfaction. Their diet becomes the catalyst for what will eventually turn into a lifetime of world-class thinking. The more fit their bodies become, the more it impacts the way they think. They realize feeling fit and full of energy is better than the best tasting unhealthy foods. They start to associate self-control and discipline with elevated feelings of happiness and well being. In the process of getting fit, they eventually reach the realization that there is no success or lasting happiness without struggle. The victory is not in the weight loss, but in the fight and inevitable triumph over oneself. So while fat people are looking for happiness in their next meal, fit people are operating from a happy mindset because they have uncovered a universal truth: sustained happiness is an inside job.

Critical Thinking Question

Would you rather experience the short term satisfaction of eating unhealthy food, or the long term pride of achieving world-class fitness?

Action Step

Take inventory of your daily actions and ask yourself if they are congruent with your personal values. If you really value fitness, does your daily compliance reflect it?

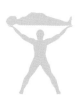

Fat people lie to themselves

Fit people are brutally honest

Fat people are liars. They work hard to convince themselves and others they don't mind being fat. Many of them have actually talked themselves into believing it. This is like failing in school and saying you're happy about it or getting fired from your job and telling people you don't care. This grand delusion is so prevalent in American society that Madison Avenue is now producing commercials promoting the idea that big is beautiful. Fat women are labeled "plus-size" to make them comfortable buying giant clothing for their bloated bodies. The underlying message is "It's OK to destroy your health and die young. . .celebrate your obesity and buy our giant clothes!" And fat people are buying it. That's the power of delusion. Fat people are starving to be told its OK to be fat so they don't have to accept personal responsibility for their failure, and advertisers are glad to assist them in this fantasy, for a hefty profit, of course. Fit people reject middle-class thinking of any kind. If they get fat, they own up to it and get busy getting thin and healthy again. They're honest with themselves. They look at their bodies with the objectivity of a stranger, and refuse to accept anything less than their best. Fit people know fat is not beautiful, but an ugly manifestation of a series of poor choices. They also know it's never too late to change, as long as the ravages of obesity and all its related diseases haven't reached the point of no return. Decide today to be brutally honest with yourself. Don't beat yourself up if you're fat. Remember that most of us have been there. Just take responsibility and fix it. In 90 days you'll be living a better life.

Critical Thinking Question

Are you being brutally honest with yourself about how you look and your current level of fitness? Can you really afford to take the weight loss/maintenance process casually? Is your life and health in danger because you're so fat?

Action Step

Grow up and get tough with yourself! You're not a kid anymore, and it's time to stop letting yourself off the hook to avoid facing reality.

Fat people don't know what they want or where they're going

Fit people have vision

The majority of people treat their bodies like rental cars. They thoughtlessly clog their arteries, poison their lungs, raise their cholesterol, and pack on extra pounds as though they can trade their body in for a new one when this model is worn out. In a society dominated by television, video games, and fast food it's easy to fall into this trap. It's not stupidity, but the lack of conscious thought. It often takes a heart attack or other major physical event to wake up to the fact that healthy eating and exercise habits cannot be ignored. Fit people are conscious of every piece of food that goes into their bodies and every act of exercise they perform. Fat people eat what tastes good and makes them feel better. Fit people eat strategically and consider the impact of every meal. The difference is rooted in the result each is after. Fat people use food to give them an emotional lift. Fit people use food to move them closer to their ultimate vision, which usually goes far beyond the taste of their dinner. Since it's well documented that fewer than 3% of people set goals, can you imagine what percentage have a detailed, written vision for their lives? The masses are living day to day in a fear based consciousness with the ultimate goal of experiencing as little pain as possible. The world class seeks achievement over comfort and is willing to fight through short term pain for long term gain. The manifestation of their vision dominates their thoughts and drives their actions. Their ultimate dream must be fulfilled, and all obstacles must give way. Start by deciding what you want and determine why you want it, especially as it relates to your health and fitness. Put it in writing and read it every day. In 90 days you'll know what it feels like to think like a fit person, and you'll never be the same. You'll eventually lose desire for foods and habits that don't move you closer to your ultimate vision.

Fat Loser Quote

❝ The middle-class has daydreams, the world-class has vision. Do you have a clearly defined vision of what you will look like at your natural weight? Are you visualizing your vision every day? This is what the great ones do. ❞

Critical Thinking Question

Do you know exactly what you want to look like? Do have you crystal clear vision of your life as a fit and healthy person?

Action Step

Invest thirty minutes today to write down exactly what you will look and feel like at your ideal weight.

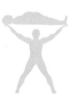

Fat people let feelings get in their way

Fit people override their emotions with logic

F at people are addicted to using food to manipulate their emotions. When they have a bad day, they know the exact foods to eat to boost their mood. When they feel sad or lonely, they know what foods alter that state of mind. Foods aren't as strong as drugs, but the emotional addiction is similar to drug addiction. Fit people rely on healthy strategies to alter their moods. The most popular among them is exercise. Fit people are great at altering negative emotions and moods by thinking about and visualizing the most exciting moments in their visions. They use logic to guide their responses to the everyday ups and down we all experience, which directs them to strategies that serve their best interests. While fat people are controlled, manipulated and bullied by their emotions, fit people rely on left-brain logic as their guide. The great ones save their emotional power to supercharge their motivation to reach their goals. They identify their emotional motivators and use them as a power tool to drive them through periods where most people give up. Emotions and feelings are powerful, but left unchecked can have disastrous effects. Seeing a tiger at the zoo is a great experience, unless the tiger is out of his cage. Imagine all that power with nothing holding it back. Feelings and emotions are just as powerful. They must be controlled, harnessed, and prepared to be utilized at the right time under the right conditions. Ignoring their influence is foolish. Start by getting them under control and substituting logic in place of emotion when making food choices. As this becomes a habit that can be managed and maintained with light discipline, the next step is to find out what motivates and excites you emotionally, and begin using this self-knowledge to drive yourself to new heights of success.

Fat Loser Quote

❝ As you fight your way through the weight loss process, you will inevitably experience feelings that threaten your focus. Don't be afraid of them, because they're a natural part of any habit change. The only thing you must adhere to without wavering is compliance to your diet. That's the key to your success. Whether you are negative or positive, feeling good or awful, or even doubting you can do it, if you stay 100% compliant you will win this fight. Mental toughness, critical thinking, and visualizing yourself at your ideal weight will make it an easier fight, but if you don't cheat you can't fail. You don't need to conquer every negative thought that crosses your mind, just conquer the thoughts that tell you to cheat. ❞

Critical Thinking Question

Are you allowing your emotions to dictate your eating and exercise behavior?

Action Step

Decide today to overrule any emotional decision that doesn't serve your best interests.

Fat people are driven by ego

Fit people are driven by spirit

During the course of our conscious day, all of us are shifting back and forth between an ego and spirit-based consciousness. The ego is fear and scarcity based, the spirit is rooted in love and abundance. As this relates to eating, the ego seeks short term pleasure and the spirit long term results. Fat people spend more time in ego and fit people more time in spirit. The fastest way to move from ego to spirit is through thoughts of gratitude. Fit people are grateful to have access to clean water, healthy foods and adequate exercise. Instead of thinking thoughts of gratitude, fat people spend much of their time feeling sorry for themselves when they can't gorge on their favorite foods like they did in the past that made them fat. They focus on thoughts of scarcity, and invest much of their mental energy wishing they could eat anything they want. They complain to themselves and others about the inconvenience of their diet and the daily burden of their exercise program. None of these thoughts are congruent with a spirit-based consciousness, which leaves them in ego much of the time. Fit people have mastered their thinking to the point that they refuse to allow ego based thoughts into their minds. Ego and spirit based thinking are both habits, and the good news is any habit can be erased and replaced with due time and diligence. Start by making a health and fitness gratitude list every morning when you wake up. Condition your mind to search for what you're grateful for in relation to food, exercise and your overall health. The list doesn't have to be long; you just need to get your mind in the habit of thinking this way. After 3-4 weeks of training, this new habit will begin to take shape and alter your unconscious thoughts. You'll start to see your health and fitness through the eyes of gratitude, which will alter your perspective forever.

❝ Beware of your ego based consciousness. Ego is stationed at a lower level of consciousness that often leads to instant gratification. The ego wants everything now, and will abandon goals, walk over other people, and exaggerate and lie if necessary to satisfy its insatiable desire. Ego will tell you to eat now and start over Monday. It will tell you to feel good even if you're not 100% compliant because at least you're doing better than you were. Ego will tell you the rules don't apply to you and you can handle a little cheating without wrecking your diet. It will tell you anything it has to in order to gain pleasure or avoid pain. Your spirit based consciousness is your higher self. This is the best of you, and where you want to reside as often as humanly possible. Your spirit will keep you on track moving toward your ultimate fitness goals. ❞

Critical Thinking Question

Is your ego interfering with your performance?

Action Step

Become more conscious of your mindset from hour to hour. Is it more ego or spirit based? The higher level of awareness you reach, the easier you will be able to make the necessary adjustments in your thinking.

Fat people don't believe integrity is related to dieting

Fit people know integrity is the most important part

Integrity is the most underrated principle in the middle-class mindset. Most people understand the role integrity plays in relationships, but fail to recognize the impact of integrity with themselves. Fat people lie to themselves and don't consider the self-destruction this creates. They plan their diet and cheat as soon as they need an emotional lift. They justify their actions by blaming other people, events, and circumstances out of their control. They know down deep they're lying to themselves but don't believe it matters. Fit people live by the law of cause and effect, which states that for every cause, there must, by law, be an effect. Breaking promises to yourself destroys your confidence and weakens your self-esteem. Fat people have lied to themselves so many times they no longer believe their own promises. This is why fat people say they will "try" to stick to their diet and "try" to exercise. Trying to do these things is how they got fat in the first place, and trying will keep them fat forever. Fit people don't try; fit people do. They know doing is the only way. This is why your success in this process is mostly about getting mentally tough enough to stick to your diet and exercise program long enough to succeed. Fit people maintain their integrity with themselves by doing what they promised they would do, no matter how tough it gets. All the positive thinking platitudes, politically correct language or outright spin will never change the fact that to be fit and healthy you must be mentally tough, and doing what you say you'll do is the heart of the process. The choice is yours: maintain self-integrity in your diet and exercise goals or die fat. It's up to you. People can support and assist you, but no one is coming to the rescue. This is a battle you must win for yourself. So make up your mind right now: what's it going to be, fit or fat? Good. Now stop talking about it and go do something to back up your promise.

Fat Loser Quote

❝ *Integrity is eating what you say you will eat. It's sticking to your exercise regimen even when you think you don't have time, or just don't feel like it. It's staying on track to become the person you know you can be. The masses think it's optional. The great ones know it's mandatory.* ❞

Critical Thinking Question

Do you have the integrity to stick to the diet and exercise goals you've set for yourself?

Action Step

Take small daily steps to build confidence in maintaining your integrity. The more often you keep your word to yourself the more trust you will build.

Fat people are ashamed to admit they're dieting

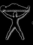

Fit people are proud of it

The masses have been conditioned to keep their dreams to themselves for fear they'll be rejected and embarrassed if they don't achieve them. Even some of the most popular psychologists in the world recommend scaling back your goals and keeping them to yourself for fear of being disappointed and humiliated. Thank God the founding fathers of America and other world-class performers never bought into that kind of middle-class thinking. The point is that even among the most educated people in the population, the fear and scarcity-based disease called middle-class thinking is alive, well, and being disseminated to the masses under the guise of emotional protection. Fat people won't admit they're dieting because of this very reason. They don't trust themselves enough to put their word on the line. Fit people tell everyone they know to create additional pressure and motivation to propel them forward when the going gets tough. They don't need to tell other people to succeed, but they use it as a tool to strengthen their mental toughness and deepen their resolve. At the highest levels, the great ones know they are role models for others who haven't tapped into their own mental toughness. They know their success will inspire others to get thin and healthy, and this becomes an additional emotional motivator. Fit people also tell others as a means of gaining support and guidance on their journey to superior fitness. Their spirit-based mindset is open to all the help and support they can get. The fact is the mentally tough thinker can do it alone if they have to, but they seek support to make the process easier. It's the tactically intelligent thing to do.

Fat Loser Quote

❝ *Discipline is the foundation of every world-class success. Without it, nothing of value would ever be achieved. Be proud to be taking control of your life and getting fit. Very few people have the guts to share their vision of success with the world, because they know they lack the mental toughness to attain it. You're different, and the ripple effect of getting thin and healthy is going to positively impact everything you do. Tell everyone you know that you're on the road to fitness and you're excited about it. There is no going back. There is no surrender. Your weight loss victory is imminent because you are unstoppable!* ❞

Critical Thinking Question

Are you keeping your diet a secret for fear of failing? Is this helping or hurting you?

Action Step

Tell five important people in your life about your diet and exercise program and give them the date you will arrive at your ideal weight. This will keep you under pressure to persist and give you the added support you'll need to make it.

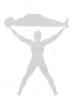

Fat people are dependent

Fit people are interdependent

As you know by now, fat thinking and middle-class thinking are synonymous. One of the foundations of both groups is their unwillingness to take responsibility for their lives. Fat people are dependent on outside forces like fad diets, weight loss drugs and new exercise routines that promise to solve their weight problem without effort or commitment. It's a mindset, a philosophy and a habitual way of thinking all rolled into one. Broke people are dependent on the government and the wealthy to rescue them. People struggling with failed relationships are dependent on marriage counselors, clergy, and psychoanalysts. Smokers are dependent on doctors to save them after a lifetime of abuse, poisoning their lungs. The list goes on and on, and it all starts with thinking. Fit people rely on themselves more than they do anyone else. They seek help, but they're not waiting for outside forces to save them. Their core belief is "I am responsible." Fit people and world-class thinkers are almost synonymous. It's not that these two groups are completely self-sufficient; no one chasing greatness ever is. But the common denominator of seeing themselves as the problem as well as the solution influences everything they do. Fit people don't eat healthy because they're so disciplined; they eat healthy because it's in their best interest. They know they are the President, CEO and Chairman of the Board of their own lives and it's their job to keep their bodies and minds functioning at their highest levels. Their philosophy of interdependence directs them to seek assistance and advice from others, but the final decision and responsibility for those decisions is always theirs. Getting thin and healthy is up to you. Getting fat is your fault, and getting thin will be your victory. Decide today to own up to these facts and then go to work to get the results you deserve.

Critical Thinking Question

Have you taken full responsibility for getting fat?
Have you taken full responsibility for getting fit?

Action Step

Accept 100% responsibility for all of your successes and failures in your life. This is the first step on the path to world-class success.

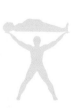

Fat people see themselves as victims

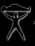

Fit people see themselves as leaders

Fit people have so much credibility with themselves they see themselves as leaders. Self-mastery is so rare that when someone achieves it in any area of his life, he is often looked up to as someone to emulate. The more people see them as leaders, the more they see themselves as leaders, and the upward spiral continues making them stronger and stronger. Fat people experience the same phenomenon in reverse. The more often they fail to commit to their diet and exercise program, the more credibility they lose with themselves. They begin to see themselves as victims. Their friends, family and members of their inner circle treat them like victims and come to expect their ongoing failure. This downward spiral further depletes their confidence until they reach the point of self-inflicted helplessness. Both the fit and fat are experiencing the same psychological and social phenomena on opposite sides, which drives the fit to get fitter and the fat, fatter. Success and failure are both self-fulfilling prophecies. What starts out as a small setback on a diet compounds into a colossal failure over time, both in the mind of the performer and the people around her. On the reverse side, what starts out as a small success on a diet eventually evolves into a massive success for the fit person. Thoughts that start out as wishful thinking soon turn into steel cables of habitual consciousness as the performer's credibility and confidence make quantum leaps in strength. It's a well known secret among world-class performers that their rapid ascension to the top is the result of a non-linear process not understood by the masses. This explains how people go from fat to fit to leader and role model in a very short time. What is impossible in the linear world is easy in the non-linear world. The key to unlocking the door and tapping into the non-linear forces is a modest but sustained success in your health and fitness. Like compound interest in wealth building, the psychological and social effects of your success create a multiplier effect in your confidence and credibility until you are seen by yourself and others as a leader in this area. And since success breeds success, (especially on the mental plane) imagine the impact this will have on every other area of your life.

Fat Loser Quote

66 *You should be the leader of your own life. Your adolescence is over, and it's time to take control. Stop buying into the messages of mediocrity handed down from so-called authority figures and start thinking for yourself. You know fat is ugly and you know it will kill you! You know better than to believe extra large clothes look sexy, or that you should just accept yourself as a fat person. You know not to judge people by their size, yet most of us do. Just because the masses can't handle the realities of life doesn't mean you have to live your life clouded by delusional thinking. Be a leader and command your mental army to boldly and bravely charge into objective reality head on and confront your challenges. When you do, you'll find the enemy isn't as tough as you thought, and that the real battle was never you against some outside force, it was you against you. This revelation will bring you full circle to realize if you can conquer yourself, you can have anything you desire. This is the hidden treasure the masses never find. It's waiting for you. Be a leader and go get it!* 99

Action Step

Decide today to become the CEO of
your own life and make your first official
action getting your body fit. This success
will fuel all future victories you'll have
as the leader of your own life.

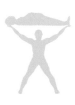

Fat people have a poor attitude toward food and exercise

Fit people have a positive attitude toward food and exercise

F at people see a healthy diet and exercise plan as something that's been forced upon them, even when they choose it themselves. They complain about how the new foods taste and go on and on about how the great the foods are that made them fat. They beg for sympathy after every workout, and long for the days of their sedentary lifestyle. Is it any wonder they end up quitting? It's like getting married and continuing to tell yourself that you don't believe in marriage and you don't love your new spouse! How many weeks would that marriage last? Fit people are in objective reality when it comes to foods that taste great but are unhealthy. They tell themselves these are the foods that made them fat and might have killed them if they didn't take action. Fit people know their attitude toward their diet and exercise program will make or break them. While fat people seek the sympathy of others, fit people seek success. Chasing sympathy is for losers! Winners don't want your sympathy, winners want to win! And winning this game means getting thin and healthy, no matter what it takes. Fit people get and stay fit by maintaining a world-class attitude, especially when they're tired and hungry. They tell themselves they are on the road to a life of abundant energy, vitality and endurance. A life of looking good and feeling good. A life feeling confident, attractive and successful. A life of being a role model for others and their children to emulate. In short, they tell themselves they are headed towards the good life. A limitless future where everything is possible. Can you see how these daily thoughts drive their success? World-class attitude is a habit you build day by day with the thoughts you think to yourself. Once you control your thoughts, you control your attitude, and ultimately, your success.

Fat Loser Quote

Approach your weight loss goal with a world-class attitude. There's no reason to make this process tougher than it is by being negative. Be excited to be on the road to a better life and grateful to have a good diet and exercise program to follow. Someone else created those tools, and all you have to do is follow them. Start seeing your diet as the opportunity of a lifetime, because that's exactly what it is. Half the world's population would do anything to trade their problems for yours. They spend their days looking for enough food to survive, and you're killing yourself through overindulgence. You have more money in your wallet than these people will earn in a lifetime, and you want to feel sorry for yourself? Wake up and gain a little perspective. Look up to the stars and thank God, or the universe, or whatever you believe in, that you only have this tiny little problem to solve. Then suck it up and get to work, and let your attitude reflect your blessings and good fortune.

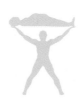

Fat people balance how poorly they can eat with how much guilt they can handle

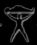

Fit people balance how healthy they can eat with how much energy they desire

The mantra of fat thinking is, "How much bad food can I get away with eating?" Fat people see food as an enemy trying to keep them fat, which leads them to be constantly thinking of ways to cheat on their diet without paying a price. Fit people see food as a tool that creates energy and vitality, which leads them to be constantly looking for healthier foods that will give them even more abundant health. Fit people believe food is a friend that's there to serve them. Not only do they enjoy the experience of eating high quality foods, but they also reap the rewards of the nutrients stored in these foods that deliver more energy, increased mental acuity and superior digestion. The fact is healthy eating makes your body function well and feel great. The better you eat the better you feel. Fat people enjoy short term satisfaction eating unhealthy foods and suffer the consequences. The only benefit eating offers them is a few minutes of fun. After each meal they feel stuffed, bloated and guilty. Fit people get a boost of confidence every time they stick their diet, which carries over into every aspect of their lives. Fit people pay the price of discipline, fat people the price of failure. Discipline must be built into a habit, but failure becomes a habit on its own. Many fat people don't realize that getting and staying fit is easier than being fat. Being fat makes you feel bad. It destroys your health, depletes your energy, and robs your self-esteem. And that's just for starters. It will infect every aspect of your life and make you believe you don't possess the power to control your own behavior. It's a snowball effect that can ruin your life. Getting and staying fit is easier, but it requires a strong commitment, especially in the first 30 days while your new habits are being formed. Take it from a former fat person: It's worth it!

Fat Loser Quote

66 *Imagine how you will feel as one of the fittest people in your family. Imagine waking up every day with an abundance of energy. Imagine feeling great about yourself and your life. This is the life that awaits you in the land of health and fitness. Balancing guilt with eating and exercise is a formula for failure, and it's the formula most people follow. If you're satisfied with settling for second best, then follow the masses and stay fat. After all, it's your life. You have the right to mediocrity and the masses will gladly you accept you. But if being fat disgusts you and the prospect of mediocrity seems like a death sentence, drop the eating/guilt habit and start eating like someone who wants to be fit. Don't you deserve to live a life of superior health and abundance? Do it now while you still have time to choose.* 99

Critical Thinking Question

Do you associate eating and exercise
more with guilt or energy?

Action Step

Start telling yourself every day that
food and exercise are for fueling your
mind and body to better assist you in
attaining your goals and dreams.

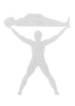

Fat people ignore the power of momentum

Fit people capitalize on the power of momentum

The concept of momentum is well understood in the physical world, but on the psychological plane, few comprehend the magnitude and raw power of a made up mind moving toward a goal and getting stronger every day. We see this phenomenon in sports, business, politics and many other areas. Fit people use momentum to propel themselves forward and reduce the resistance they experience from the old habits trying to hang on. Old eating habits can be painful to break in the beginning, but once you make it through the first week or so, psychological momentum kicks in and you start to believe you will succeed. Then you start to lose weight, and the momentum gets even stronger. Next, people start to notice and comment on how good you look, which builds even more momentum. And it just gets stronger every day. The stronger the momentum gets, the easier it is to stick to your diet and exercise program. What other people see as discipline is really just an attempt to keep the momentum growing as you get thinner and healthier every day. Fit people know the hardest part of building momentum is getting started. Fat people look in the mirror and are overwhelmed with the amount of weight they must lose, because they're thinking in linear fashion. Fit people know after the first week or so, momentum will kick in and sticking to the diet will get easier and easier. Momentum takes something linear and makes it non-linear through the magic of the mind. Psychological momentum cannot be quantified, but it can be experienced. And since getting and staying fit is an emotional process, it's something you must master.

Fat Loser Quote

❝ *Human beings are emotional creatures that have the ability to thrive off of psychological momentum. The more fit you get, the more excited you become. The more compliments you receive. The more eyes you feel looking at you. And the momentum builds exponentially like a snowball thundering down a mountain. During the first days of your weight loss, the pain you experience will be linear to your results, but as momentum kicks in you will feel less pain and more excitement with every pound you lose. Most people don't stick to their diet long enough to experience this phenomenon. Just be patient and compliant and the "Big Mo" will kick in and eventually gain hurricane-like force and carry you to the finish line. You are about to go on the ride of your life. Your only ticket to entry is 100% compliance. Everything else will be taken care of whether you believe it or not. Just stick to your diet and exercise program and let momentum take care of the rest.* ❞

Critical Thinking Question

Are you building more momentum every
day by staying 100% compliant with
your diet and exercise program?

Action Step

Harness the power of momentum today by doing
exactly what you promised yourself you would do.

Fat people silently suffer the consequences of failure

Fit people build a team to help them succeed

It's not easy being fat. As a matter of fact, it sucks. After two years of being 40 pounds overweight, I can say with authority it was not a pleasant experience. Fat people suffer in many ways, and much of the suffering is done alone. Being fat is a private failure you share with the public. It's the first thing people notice when you meet. It's like wearing a sign around your neck that says, "Yes, I'm fat and failing in this area of my life." You can't hide fat, and there's nothing good about it. It's ugly, uncomfortable and unattractive. It's also deadly. Walking around fat is like being broke and everyone you meet knows it instantly. Fat people silently suffer physically, psychologically, and socially. Fit people have the opposite experience. They're praised and respected for their success, especially in a world full of plump people. Fit people are seen as more disciplined, organized and successful. And that's before they even utter a word! World-class thinkers who decide to get fit build a team of people to help them end their suffering. This team may include a personal trainer, nutritionist and coach, or it may just be a group of family and friends to help support their efforts and sustain their motivation. So while fat people quietly suffer, fit people share their journey with a team of people committed to keeping them on track until they succeed. And since weight is hard to hide, the team knows if you are winning or not. Within a matter of weeks, the weight drops, exercise increases, new eating and exercise habits are forming, and the team showers the performer with love and praise. It's easy to quit when you're on your own, but letting down a team of people who care about you is a different story. Building a team is one of the great secrets of world-class performers.

Fat Loser Quote

66 *Smart people don't attempt any goal of substantial proportion alone. Habit change may be simple, but it's certainly not easy. Assemble a mentor and support team to guide and encourage you along your journey. The self-made man/woman approach is more about ego than intelligent strategy, and should be avoided at all costs. Allow your spirit-based consciousness to guide you in selecting your success team, and then go build it person by person.* 99

Critical Thinking Question

Do you have a support team in place to help you through the tough times of habit change?

Action Step

Contact three of your closest friends and family members today and ask them to be on your support team.

Fat people believe the thinking that made them fat will make them thin

Fit people know if they want to succeed they have to change

Fat people aren't fat because they're undisciplined. They're not fat because they have low self-esteem. And they're not fat because they are missing anything. Fat people are fat because they think fat. In other words, their thoughts and philosophies direct them to behave in ways that make them fat. They see French fries, onion rings and pizza and think, "yum!" Fit people see these foods and think, "poison." The food is the same, only the thoughts are different. So the fat person eats the bad foods and the fit person walks away. Fat thinking will not make you fit. Only fit thinking will work. If you're fat and you want to be fit, you need to change your thinking. Be aware that fit thinkers are a small minority, and prepare for a push back from your fat thinking family and friends. Not knowing they're hurting you, they will attempt to pull you back to fat thinking. This is not for you. Stick close to your team and confide in them when you feel weak, but never give in. This is a fight you must win, and it's not going away, nor will it get any easier. If you allow yourself to be sucked back into fat thinking, you will eventually die fat. And the saddest part is, it will be your own fault. The purpose of this book is for you to learn how fit people think and encourage you to copy their thought processes, habits and philosophies. Once you build the habit of thinking like a fit person, your life will change forever in ways you can't imagine. I've never seen anything like it the arena of personal growth. As a mental toughness coach, I've helped people make more money, have better relationships, communicate more effectively, and a host of other things, but I've never seen a more dramatic impact on a human being than their journey from fat to fit. It gives you confidence money can't buy, and you carry that confidence into every aspect of your existence. Without exaggeration, the benefits of getting fit are almost impossible to overstate.

Fat Loser Quote

66 *Thinking like a broke person will keep you broke. Thinking like an unhappy person will keep you unhappy. Thinking like a fat person will keep you fat. Fat is just the effect, thinking is the cause. Think like a fit person and you'll behave in ways that make you fit. Most people are focused on changing the effect, but the secret is changing the cause, and the effect will take care of itself.* 99

Critical Thinking Question

Are you really prepared to change your thinking about diet and exercise?

Action Step

Start repeating this phrase to yourself every day: "I think like a fit person" Say this to yourself and everyone around you until it's hardwired into your belief system.

Fat people allow failures of the past to hold them back

Fit people use failure to move forward

One of the thought patterns fat people fall into is assuming their future will be the same as their past. They've tried dozens of diets, lost weight and gained it back. They started to exercise, then got out of the habit and went back to their old ways. They wallow in their feelings of failure and are reluctant to commit to another diet, believing it will be a replay of the past. The fact is, everyone on earth has failed at something. Many of us multiple times. You are not alone. The difference is, fit people know the past doesn't equal the future, and they take the same failures as fat people and use them to propel themselves toward success. They know how bad being fat feels, and they decide they never want to experience that pain again. Every time they feel like cheating, they remember how it felt when they quit their last diet and the secret shame they silently suffered. Fat people see unhealthy foods and remember what eating them in the past did to their body. They recall being bloated, stuffed, and uncomfortable and they don't want to feel that way ever again. Fat people depress themselves remembering their failures, while fit people excite themselves imagining how it will feel when they hit their ideal weight. The past can't be changed, but the way we perceive it can. It's in your control. It's up to you. Using past failures as a motivator isn't popular with the masses, so don't expect to tell people about this and receive universal praise. Remember, the majority of the population falls into middle-class thinking, which means they get pleasure from being a victim. Only a small percentage of the population embraces world-class thinking, and fit people are among them. Decide today you will be one of them, and ignore the beliefs and philosophies of middle-class mediocrity. There's a bright new future out there waiting for you. All you have to do is claim it and your life will change. You can do it!

Fat Loser Quote

66 *The masses see failure as further proof that they're not good enough, educated enough, or smart enough to get what they want. World-class performers see failure as a learning experience that allows them to start over at a higher level of awareness. It's not that they enjoy failing, but instead of proof of their incompetence, they see it as proof of their persistence. The failure event is the same for both groups, but the interpretation of its meaning is 180 degrees different. This perceptual shift is one of the mental toughness secrets of the great ones, and you can adopt it immediately by simply redefining what failure means to you.* 99

Critical Thinking Question

Do you believe it's possible to use your failures
of the past as a springboard for future success?

Action Step

Decide today to let go of the fear of
failing on your diet and move forward with the
self-assurance of a champion.
Remember your success in this process is
completely up to you. Just for today, act like it's
impossible to fail, and experience what it's like
to live your life with world-class confidence.

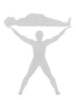

Fat people are unaware of the opportunity getting fit presents

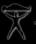

Fit people seize the opportunities fitness offers

Fat people who have never lived in a fit body have no idea what they're missing. They have no idea what it's like to have a body with boundless energy and endless stamina. If they had any clue of the beautiful life getting fit offers, they would begin a world-class diet immediately and access every ounce of mental toughness necessary to make it successful. Fit people have experienced the full benefits fitness presents, spanning the spectrum of physical, mental and spiritual. If they lose focus and gain weight, they quickly get back on track. This isn't because they're so disciplined, but because they have personally experienced the vast array of opportunities fitness offers. People do judge a book by its cover, and a fit body shows the world you have mastered this critical area of your life and gives them confidence you are capable of conquering challenges. Fat people don't get second looks from people of the opposite sex, but fit people get noticed. Fat people applying for jobs are often discriminated against, while fit people are seen as more organized, competent and in control of their lives. Fat people have a strike against them in business dealing with suppliers, customers and co-workers, while fit people have a distinct advantage. Fat people are poor role models for their children in the area of health and fitness. Kids of fat parents get the message it's OK to be fat, and that fitness should not be a priority. Fit parents are setting an example for their kids without saying a word. The benefits and opportunities of fitness are too numerous to list and must be experienced to be appreciated. Haven't you heard enough to go for it? Come on, take a chance on yourself! You are tougher than you think.

Fat Loser Quote

66 *Getting fit is arguably the single greatest opportunity any of us will ever have during the course of our lives. The aggregate effect of succeeding at something most people fail at is hard to overstate. Waking up every day looking good, feeling good, and basking in uncommon success is a daily injection of confidence, self-esteem and well being. And this all occurs during the first 30 seconds of the day! Imagine starting every day with this type of feeling. You carry that confidence into everything you do and everyone you come into contact with. The ripple effect of fitness touches every aspect of your life in a positive way. Can you really afford to treat this process like a hobby?* 99

Critical Thinking Question

Are you aware of how many benefits are waiting for you when you achieve your fitness goal? Do you understand that this is going to alter the course of your entire life and become one of the most important things you'll ever do?

Action Step

Contact someone who is really fit and ask them what it's like to live in a thin and healthy body. You'll be overwhelmed at his or her response.

Fat people are mentally unorganized

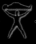

Fit people use mental organization to stay thin and healthy

When it comes to diet and exercise, fat people are either uncommitted or mentally unorganized. Much of a healthy diet consists of proper planning and effective strategy. Fat people eat what they like and what's convenient, whether it's in their best interests or not. Fit people are master planners and rarely eat foods not on their plan. They develop exercise programs that maximize their dieting efforts and follow them religiously. Fit people seek help from diet and exercise coaches and mentors if they believe it will help them. They know what's at stake, and refuse to allow ego to get in the way. Fit people know poor planning is a recipe for dieting disaster, especially during times of high emotion, late night fatigue, and social pressure during holidays and special occasions. This planning covers everything from stocking healthy foods, packing nutritionally sound snacks, and coordinating travel plans with healthy restaurants and hotels that offer adequate exercise facilities. Fit people are mentally prepared for the temptations they will encounter along their journey, such as negative friends and family. They know the pitfalls of middle-class thinking, and are ready to ignore this self-destructive mindset. This includes the assault of the media that pushes the idea we should all accept our bodies as they are, because fat is beautiful. Fit people know this philosophy is the epitome of middle-class thinking and they reject it. Fat people are more susceptible to these types of messages because they're not mentally prepared for them. The message is clear: get organized in every way possible and be prepared for the mental and physical obstacles you will surely encounter.

Fat Loser Quote

Critical Thinking Question

Are you as organized in your diet and exercise program as you need to be to stay on course?

Action Step

Map out your eating and exercising plan of action every night before you go to bed to be sure you're properly prepared for the next day.

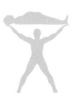

Fat people are stressed

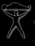

Fit people are at peace with themselves

F at people see fit people and wonder how they discipline themselves to maintain their beautiful bodies. Fit people look at fat people and wonder how they are mentally tough enough to endure the pain and suffering of being fat yet fail to transfer their toughness to getting fit. The truth is, fat people experience far more stress, anxiety and pain than fit people by the physical and mental burden of their failure. As their health declines, their stress and anxiety increase, exacerbating the issue. Fit people enjoy the pride, joy, and peace of mind that accompanies success. They wake in the morning with superior energy, and the mindset of a winner. When they look in the mirror, they see the results of their success, achievement, discipline, planning, and most of all, their mental toughness. This ongoing emotional satisfaction and fulfillment accompanies them all day long, and gives them a boost of energy. This gives them an edge on their competition in the workplace. Their peace of mind carries over into their relationships and every other facet of their lives. While fat people sink deeper into depression over their failure, fit people are emboldened by their success. If fat people only understood the price they're paying for failure is much higher than the price of success, they would get thin and healthy, wouldn't they? If you're reading this and saying it can't be this simple, you're wrong. Getting fit is simple, but not easy. Not in the beginning, anyway. My point is that compared with the physical, mental and spiritual torture you have to endure as a fat person, getting fit is a bargain! Suffering for the sake of suffering is stupid. The good news is, you are only one decision away from changing your life. Are you ready to make a commitment, or do I need to make a stronger case?

Fat Loser Quote

❝ *The stress of being fat is enough to kill you. The emotional suffering that accompanies excessive weight is enough to destroy anyone's self-esteem. The physical, mental and emotional price people pay for being fat is astronomical, especially when you factor in how simple getting fit can be. Sure, you have to be mentally tough to succeed, but nowhere near as tough as you have to be in order to live with being fat. Fit people live in a peaceful and harmonious state of mind and ride the wave of momentum being fit generates. Being fit is a natural state that allows your body to operate at its potential, which subsequently affects your thoughts and feelings about everything. Getting fit is one the most effective stress reduction strategies you will ever employ.* ❞

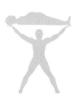

Fat people quit easily

Fit people employ the power of persistence

The masses are mired in microwave mentality, which demands instant results for ongoing effort. Whether it's getting fit, making money or building a better marriage, middle-class thinking is a formula for losing. It's the reason so many smart people with limitless talent are fat, broke and frustrated with their lot in life. Fit people know middle-class thinking is the disease, and world-class thinking is the cure. One of the most overlooked and underrated secrets of great performers is persistence. Fit people know there's no magic to being fit, but it does require persistent action whether the results are obvious or not. The ability to hang on in the face of discouragement, fatigue, and hunger is critical to getting fit. The good news is the toughest part of the process only lasts a few weeks, when the new habits begin to take root. The load is lightened within 7-10 days as the weight starts to come off. That strengthens the performers resolve to stay committed. Fat people have given up too early so many times it's become habitual. When they lose weight they usually gain it back by slipping back into their old ways of thinking. Their lack of persistence carries over from the physical to the mental, and they allow the thoughts that made them fat to creep back into their consciousness Fit people thoroughly understand the role persistence plays on both the physical and mental planes. They are aware that persistent middle-class thinking will make them fat while persistent world-class thinking will make them thin. Our bodies are the physical manifestation of our thinking around food and exercise. Fit people persistently have thoughts that dictate behaviors that move them closer to their fitness goals every day. They know a world-class habit of thought can be unraveled by middle-class thinking in a very short period of time, and they remain militant to make sure it doesn't happen. We all apply persistence to paying our bills, brushing our teeth, and taking regular showers, so why can't we apply this same level of persistence to monitoring our thoughts?

Fat Loser Quote

66 *One of the largest gaps between the middle class and world class is in their capacity to persist. The masses are famous for their inability to discipline themselves to hang on when the going gets tough. They'll persist through the ongoing suffering of mediocre results, but are seemingly blind to the fact that the same persistence applied to success would get them everything they ever dreamed of. The breakdown occurs because most people never transcend the level of consciousness that created the problem in the first place. The great ones know that a problem cannot be solved at the same level of consciousness in which it occurred, so their first step is raising their level of thinking, usually by copying the thought patterns and philosophies of people who are succeeding. In the land of world-class thinking, persistence is king.* 99

Critical Thinking Question

Are you committed to persist on
your diet until you succeed?

Action Step

Identify five different times in your life
when you persisted until you succeeded,
and write them down.
Read them every morning for the next
seven days and immerse yourself in the
consciousness it took to persevere.

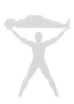

Fat people feel powerless to change

Fit people believe they can do anything

Fat people become obese when they lose faith in their ability to change. Failure after failure feeds on itself and turns into a psychological tempest that seems insurmountable to the middle-class mindset. To ease the pain of failure they eat until their very existence is at stake. They sink deeper into depression and despair with each passing day as their health deteriorates in front of their eyes. Adding to their misery is the fact their failure is on display for the world to see, which creates feelings of shame, worthlessness, and self-loathing. Fat people eventually experience 'conditioned powerlessness', a mindset in which they feel they are victims of an outside force they cannot overcome. Fit people know personal power is just a perception controlled by the individual. They understand past failures, no matter how numerous, have nothing to do with future success. Fit people have mastered the art of decision making, and the mental toughness to stick to their decisions. While fat people look at 100 pounds of fat as an insurmountable obstacle, fit people see it as a process of losing 1 pound 100 times. They reduce the size and scope of the task by breaking it down into 'believable losses.' Fit people avoid the downward psychological spiral of despair and depression by letting go of past failures and focusing 100% of their mental energy on the beautiful future they have envisioned. They tap their personal power during meal choices until healthy eating is a habit. They use their power to motivate themselves to exercise when they're tired and hungry. While fat people seek sympathy for their struggle from middle-class thinkers, fit people keep their own counsel and tap into their mentor and support teams for further advice. They've learned thinking like a fat person is what makes you fat, and they refuse to take advice from other fat people in this area. Your mental power can be used any way you choose. Maybe it's time to start directing your mind in ways that help you rather than hurt you?

Fat Loser Quote

❝ You are now at a crossroads in your life. You can go down the fat road or the fit road. The fat road leads to feelings of failure, depression and despair. The fit road leads to feelings of success, joy and pride. The fat road requires no toll. The fit road requires 21-30 days of discipline while you upgrade your habits. You are the only one who can decide which way to go. Which road will you take? ❞

Critical Thinking Question

Do you really want to go back to the days
of feeling guilty about what you eat and
watching your body expand by the day? Is
eating unhealthy foods really worth having
to endure feelings of depression, despair
and self-loathing for the rest of your life?

Action Step

Start telling yourself everyday that
you can do anything you decide to do.
Begin encouraging others by telling them
the same thing about themselves and
you'll start to build positive momentum
in this area. The more you repeat this
phrase, the more you will believe it.

Fat people negotiate the price of success

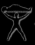

Fit people pay the price

Fat people diet like just as you'd suspect: like it's a light undertaking they're playing around with. Fat people are always cutting back by not having dessert, pushing aside the mashed potatoes, or sending the bread back to the kitchen. Their delusional thinking tells them these small, yet non-strategic actions will make them healthy. And when they weigh the same or more day after day, they're confounded by their failure. The real problem is, fat people think getting fit is negotiable. They treat it like a game, going off their diet every weekend, holiday and special occasion while promising to start over again on Monday. This failure pattern is easily detected by objective outsiders, yet it remains a mystery to the fat person with her eyes wide shut. Fit people know getting fit is simple and straightforward, yet absolutely non-negotiable. You eat healthy and exercise consistently according to the guidelines of a successful diet or you will eventually die fat. Fat people like to make this simple process as complex and full of mystery as possible to support their belief that being fat is not their fault. Of course, the fact is, it is their fault, as well as their responsibility to get fit. In other words, if I tell myself and others how complicated it is to travel from point A to point B, the more excuses I can make for taking detours and failing to make the trip. The scary thing is that much of this middle-class thinking occurs at the unconscious level, proving the raw power of psychological self-delusion. People are capable of talking themselves into almost anything. If you think I'm exaggerating the power of self-delusion, consider this gruesome fact: Thousands of German soldiers facilitated the slaughter of six million innocent men, women and children whose only crime was being of Jewish descent, during World War II. Were these men really evil, or were they conditioned to believe they were doing the right thing? How could any human being participate in the mass extermination of innocent people? This mentality is no different than today's suicide bombers. Psychological conditioning by themselves and others leads the way, and their actions are justified by delusional thinking. When you put it into perspective, believing that delusion keeps people fat is not that big of a stretch. Decide to keep it simple and pay the price to get fit. If you fail, accept full responsibility and start over. Keep in mind that fat people suffer every day while fit people only suffer for a few weeks during the new habit incubation period. There's no comparison when it comes to which group pays the higher price.

Fat Loser Quote

❝ *Most people who fail to get fit aren't weak, they're just delusional. They honestly believe they can negotiate the price of success. They stick to their diet during the week, and cheat on the weekends, all the while believing they will still lose weight. Never underestimate the power of self-delusion. It's alive and well in fat people who believe 99% compliance is A+ work. Wouldn't it be easier to just pay the price and end this nightmare once and for all? If getting fit was really negotiable, wouldn't fewer people be fat?* ❞

Critical Thinking Question

Are you wasting your mental energy
on creative ways to negotiate the price
of your fitness, or investing it in solving
this problem once and for all?

Action Step

Realize that you can't negotiate your way
out of this. You must pay the price, and
the longer you wait the higher it will be.
Decide today to get it done and move past
this irritating plague of the masses.

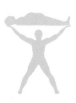

Fat people fail to prepare

Fit people prepare to win

Proper preparation is a necessity in the weight loss process, especially in the first 30 days when the new habits are being formed. Healthy meals need to be planned in advance of getting hungry, exercise needs to be scheduled before fatigue sets in, and the proper mindset must be chosen in advance of the psychological struggle of habit change. No war is fought before a battle plan is established and the consequences of prepared actions are estimated. Getting fit is simple, but not easy, at least not in the beginning while the old habits are still strong. Fit people pack healthy foods when they travel, set their exercise routine in advance, and mentally prepare themselves for the experience of physical and psychological change. All that's left is execution and the mental toughness to ride the storm out. Fat people love to deny that the battle of the bulge is a battle. They still believe they can make a few small changes and someday wake up thin and healthy. The truth is if they don't win the war they will die fat, and their premature death may even be caused by the fat they treated like a friend. When countries invade other countries, their political propaganda machine often refers to it as 'military procedure' or a 'temporary occupation'. You can spin it any way you want, but it's still a war. The battle of the bulge is a psychological war you fight from the inside. It's the new habits versus the old established habits, and it can get downright uncomfortable. The old habits have the bigger, stronger, more established army. The new habits only have a dream of a better life and the hope of pulling an upset. It's not an easy fight, but it is winnable. By admitting you're in a tough psychological war you are mentally preparing yourself for battle and won't be surprised when doubt, fear and fatigue start knocking at your door telling you to give up. Fit people are afraid to acknowledge that getting thin and healthy is a tough fight against strong opponent. Just by acknowledging this fact, it automatically reduces the intimidation of being the underdog. After all, if getting fit was so easy, why are there so many fat people? Do you really believe people when they say they don't mind being fat? What they are really saying is, they've reconciled themselves to the fact that they've lost the war and resigned their fate. Fat people call that acceptance. Fit people call it surrender. Your commitment to world-class physical, mental and emotional preparation will make or break you in this process.

Fat Loser Quote

66 *Everyone wants to be fit, but only the truly committed are willing to prepare to be fit. People marvel at professional boxers who are so fit they can fight at full strength for 45 minutes. But the more impressive fact is these boxers train for 45,000 minutes to prepare for a 45 minute fight. No crowd, no reporters, no TV cameras. Much of this 45,000 minutes is done in solitude. The preparatory phase is 99% of the process, yet very few fans ever witness it. The fighter knows without this preparation he has no chance. Getting fit is less extreme, but no different. You prepare to win or you will fail.* 99

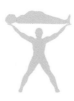

Fat people see weight management as a chore

Fit people see it as personal development

Fat people dread dieting because they anticipate pain. Getting fit is something to be put off for another day which never arrives. Fit people are aware of the far reaching benefits of physical fitness. They know if they can master their body, they can master anything. Getting fit is a life changing process and personal development course rolled into one. So while it's not easy, it offers so many rewards for success, it's crazy for anyone to refuse the challenge. If fat people understood this they wouldn't be fat! As critical as getting thin and healthy is to ones physical health, the psychological benefits may be even more significant. Getting fit is life changing. Fat people who get fit through mental toughness are never the same. They make more money, take more risks, assert themselves more often and attract what they want. The catalyst to this metamorphosis is the self-confidence a person develops by winning this very personal, internal battle. Once this new level of confidence is established, it paves the way for additional world-class beliefs. So while fat people think getting fit is only about getting physically healthy and looking better, fit people know it's also about expanding one's belief system to the point where they realize anything is possible. If you've been fit in the past, you already know this. If not, you will experience it soon enough. This is the truth about what's at stake. Now you know why this is a war you must win!

Fat Loser Quote

Fit people are more successful, more fulfilled and happier than fat people. Fit people make more money, enjoy healthier relationships and feel better about themselves than fat people. Is overeating really worth giving up all the good things in life?

Critical Thinking Question

Have you fully considered the impact getting fit will have on all aspects of your life?

Action Step

Write down the five most important characteristics of highly successful people and ask yourself this question: would getting fit give me all five?

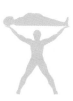

Fat people wallow in their problem

Fit people solve their problem

Fat people spend a lot of time thinking about how they got fat, how bad they feel about themselves and what they should do about it. They invest a significant amount of mental energy wallowing in the problem and very little solving it. The truth is, solving it only requires a simple decision to do whatever it takes to get fit. Little thought is needed on the part of the dieter, because the creators of the diets have done all the technical work. There's a health club on every street corner, personal trainers to assist you, and more information about how to exercise at home or on the road than ever before. The truth is, dieting and exercise no longer require much thought. There are numerous world-class diets to follow. The only part of the equation you have to master is the mental toughness to stick to your decision. Fit people know this, and invest a lot of their mental energy in tools that help them stay tough and succeed. The personal development movement was founded by people who understood the power of a made up mind, and fit people from all walks of life have tapped into the numerous authors, speakers, and unique thinkers who lead this industry. Middle-class thinkers criticize the self-help industry for being overly enthusiastic, ambitious, and optimistic, while world-class thinkers have locked into their ideas, philosophies and energy. Whether it's reading a chapter a day in Napoleon Hill's "Think and Grow Rich," or watching a DVD of Brian Tracy, fit people immerse themselves in the world of success and achievement. This immersion helps them stay mentally tough and on track toward their fitness goal. Each day they get stronger, tougher, and more focused.

Critical Thinking Question

Have you made iron clad decision to succeed on your diet no matter what it takes?

Action Step

For the next 24 hours, refuse to allow yourself to wallow in the past and instead focus on the future.

Fat people focus on pain

Fit people focus on results

Fat people choose to stay fat because they fear the pain of following a healthy diet. It's a choice between what they perceive as the lesser of two evils: being fat and dieting. The truth is, fat people only experience significant suffering in the dieting process when they haven't made a decision to succeed. Playing with a diet is like playing with a rattlesnake. It's a bad idea. Getting thin and healthy is an all or nothing process. You're either 100% committed or you're not. 99% compliance is unacceptable. Fit people know this and focus their mental energy on results. They spend very little time thinking about the pain of making a lifestyle change because it's not in their best interests. This is no different than other areas of life. Unhappy people focus on what's missing in their life, happy people focus on what they're grateful for. Broke people focus on not having enough money, rich people focus on creating more abundance. People who experience ongoing relationship problems focus on other people's flaws, people with healthy relationships focus on the positive traits of others. See the pattern, here? Many people are confounded by their results, but the root cause always begins with thinking. The good news is we have complete control of how we think and the power to change our thoughts and perceptions at any time. The only downside of this belief is the relinquishing of the right to blame anyone else for future failures. If you accept the idea that you have the power to change your life by changing your thinking, you automatically accept full responsibility for your results. This is a trade off most middle-class thinkers are not willing to make. The prospect of having no one to blame is too daunting to consider. The masses get an emotional/ psychological benefit from the sympathy they receive from others when they portray themselves as a victim. It takes more guts to succeed than it does to give up and blame the diet, exercise program, or your spouse for not being supportive. Fit people are committed, unafraid of success, and willing to bet on themselves, even if no one else is. It all starts with where they choose to focus their mental energy.

Fat Loser Quote

66 *Direct your mental energy toward the image of your body exactly the way you want to see it. Redirect any thoughts of self-pity, fatigue or sacrifice toward seeing your success in the mirror. Fat people allow their thoughts to wander, like a pinball bouncing from bumper to bumper, and their thoughts end up clinging to the old patterns that have kept them fat. In order to break this failure cycle, you must consciously control your thoughts until new patterns are ingrained enough to take over. It's a psychological tug of war for 21-30 days, but once the new pathways are created it gets easier. The pain you're experiencing in the change process is the key to your success. Embrace it and be grateful for the opportunity it presents.* 99

Critical Thinking Question

During the course of your day, what percentage of your mental energy is being directed towards the struggle of the weight loss process, compared to the percentage directed towards the results you're expecting?

Action Step

Starting today, begin to consciously control and direct your mental energy to thoughts of love, abundance, gratitude and success, and redirect thoughts of struggle and pain.

Fat people blame outside circumstances for their failure

Fit people take responsibility

A billion dollar industry has been built around the premise that diets don't work and getting fat isn't your fault. Marketers are acutely aware of how delusional the masses are about why they're failing in this area. The middle-class mindset can't handle the psychological impact of taking responsibility for their results. It's just too much for them to bear. That's why the marketers of so-called magic weight loss pills, potions, formulas, and exercise routines all claim to be the missing link. They're capitalizing on the delusional thinking of millions of people and making a fortune. Fit people are grounded in objective reality. They know getting fat is their fault, and they accept full responsibility. They know there are only two possible solutions to the problem: the first one is to make a decision to change their diet and exercise habits and get thin and healthy, and the second one is to stay fat and stop struggling. Those are the only two intelligent choices, because making a half commitment is psychological torture. You don't get to eat what you want and you don't lose weight. There's no benefit, yet it's the most common approach of the masses. This is easy to prove since most people don't succeed on diets. Is it the diet that's failing these people or their inability to stick to it? The other choice is to stay fat and continue berating yourself about it. Again, mental torture with no benefit, but shockingly, many people choose this path. Since health and fitness is vital to our very survival, the only real choice is to solve this problem once and for all. Do what fit people do: change your diet and exercise habits, drop the extra weight, and get thin and healthy. Decide to get tough with yourself and take responsibility. I promise you that not only will you feel better and live longer, it will have a massive impact on every other area of your life.

Fat Loser Quote

66 *You're in total control of your fitness. You made yourself fat, and you can make yourself thin. If you're willing to settle for a mediocre existence you can blame anyone you want for your failure. But if you want to manifest your potential, wake up and realize you are the problem and you are the solution. The masses expend huge amounts of mental energy looking for someone or something to blame. You can use that same energy to succeed. Make a pledge to yourself that you'll never blame anyone or anything for your setbacks and failures in life. Always track it back to you. This puts you in 100% control of your life. This is one of the most important mental toughness secrets of the world class.* 99

Critical Thinking Question

Are you still blaming outside circumstances or other people for your fat problem, or have you grown up and accepted the fact that you're fat and it's all your fault?

Action Step

Decide today to release any middle class or adolescent beliefs you've been holding onto, and replace them with world class and adult beliefs, the heart of which are rooted in personal responsibility.

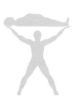

Fat people are trapped in adolescent thinking

Fit people grow up and get tough with themselves

Middle-class thinking is the psychological disease of the masses, which holds them back from realizing their full potential. The middle-class mindset is rooted in adolescent thinking, a phenomenon that occurs when adults don't expand their beliefs, philosophies and behaviors beyond what they learned as teenagers. Most of us were raised by parents, taught by teachers, and trained by coaches who were well-intentioned middle-class thinkers. They gave us everything they had, but they couldn't give us something they didn't have: world-class thinking. Fit people know that while others were responsible for building our belief system as children, we are responsible for our own psychological evolution. Fit people grow up emotionally and get tough with themselves. They wake up to the fact that once you have a diet and exercise plan, getting fit comes down to discipline, persistence and willpower. Nothing more, nothing less. And while the media and corporate profiteers love to deny the truth of this statement, world-class thinkers know their message is directed toward the masses that are too weak to handle objective reality. Once you begin holding yourself accountable for your level of fitness, everything changes. You begin ignoring mass-directed messages and following the philosophies of people getting results. Fat people who adopt these ideas and get fit are always shocked at how little time it takes to move from fit to fat. The most frequent comment we receive at the Fat Losers program from successful students is "I should have done this years ago". The biggest struggle for most fat people is making a decision to get fit. Once the commitment is made, physical, mental and spiritual forces seem to come to your aid, and everything falls into place. Whether it's psychological, spiritual or simply the momentum generated by the power of a made up mind, most people are pleasantly surprised by the experience. The key is, your decision must be solid. You must commit to do whatever it takes to succeed.

Fat Loser Quote

Now is the time to grow up and get tough with yourself. Many people would gladly trade their problems for yours. Getting fit is like taking a vacation compared to living among poverty, famine and war. Be grateful to have the opportunity to optimize your health. Most of the world would do anything to have the same chance.

Critical Thinking Question

When it comes to dieting, exercise, fat and fitness, is your thinking grounded in the objective reality of an adult or the self-delusion of a child?

Action Step

Do you still believe these five major adolescent delusions about diet and exercise?
1. Diets don't work
2. I'm obese but healthy
3. Getting fat isn't my fault
4. I'm only a few pounds overweight
5. I don't have time to exercise

Fat people suffer from low self-esteem

Fit people think highly of themselves

Being fat wreaks havoc on how you feel about yourself. Waking up every day and staring in the mirror at a bloated, distorted, overfed and under exercised body doesn't foster positive feelings. Even the movement by mental health professionals to encourage fat people to accept themselves doesn't eliminate the psychological destruction. Resigning yourself to a life of obesity, disease and early death is weak, stupid, and unnecessary. Getting fit may not be easy, but anyone can do it with mental toughness. All of us have disciplined ourselves to succeed in one area or another, so the concept is nothing new. Fit people tap into world-class thinking and throw caution to the wind. They ignore the middle-class idea that 'big is beautiful' and we should accept ourselves no matter how fat and unhealthy we are. World-class thinking won't allow them to settle for a life of mediocrity, Instead, it demands that they stay grounded in a love and abundance mindset that looks past the obstacles and focuses on the opportunities. While fat people are complaining about the discipline of dieting, fit people are moving towards their ideal weight with enthusiasm. Their self-esteem grows with every pound they lose, and creates a psychological compounding effect that makes them more mentally tough every day. The physical aspect of losing weight is a linear process, but the mental aspect is non-linear. Once the decision is made, the mental energy required to harness the fear of failing is re-directed toward strategies to succeed. The most mentally taxing part of the process occurs before the change in habits even begins. Once the decision is made, psychological momentum begins to weave its magic through the process of lightening the load. If fat people knew this they probably wouldn't hesitate to get started. The truth is most of them have failed in the past because they decided to 'try' to change their habits instead of making a serious commitment. People who 'try' to get fit stop trying when they get hungry, tired, or stressed. People who make serious commitments persist until they succeed.

Fat Loser Quote

66 *The cost of low self-esteem is substantial. Being fat is like wearing a kick me sign on your back. People see you as out of control, and you know they're right. The good news is high self-esteem is right around the corner. Walking around with a fit body people notice is an amazing elixir everyone who pays the price deserves to experience. The worse the obesity epidemic gets, the more your level of fitness stands out. While self-esteem is definitely an inside job, it sure helps to accelerate the process with the ongoing encouragement of other people.* 99

Action Step

Begin repeating this statement to
yourself and others: "compliance is
the key to fitness." If you stay 100%
compliant on your diet and exercise program,
your success is guaranteed. Program this
statement into your consciousness and
it will assist you in making it a fact.

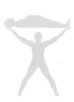

Fat people underestimate the power of energy

Fit people elevate their rate of vibration

Nothing drains energy like being fat. If it were just a matter of physical energy, it would be tolerable, but the devastating effects on a fat person's mental, emotional and spiritual energy cannot be overstated. The looks of disgust from other people. The discrimination and judgments. The automatic assumption that you have no self-discipline or willpower. These are just a few of the daily negative inputs that deplete a fat person's energy. The sad fact is, it has become so common it no longer shocks anyone. This is why I chose to be so direct with you in this book. Through kindness and an attempt to be politically correct, society has enabled millions of people to destroy their health through bad habits. The purpose of my direct approach is not to be mean, but to shock fat people back into the reality that being fat is slowing killing them. There is nothing good about being fat. Physically, emotionally, mentally and spiritually it will cause you nothing but problems and pain. Everyone knows this, but in an effort to be politically correct, society has softened the language and labels for fat people. Unfortunately, our good intentions have created a society of people who think being fat is acceptable. History has proven the majority of people are followers, and through social tolerance we have led fat people straight to a life of low energy, diminished vitality and an early grave. Fit people know this and choose to raise their vibratory rate to the highest level possible to keep them on track and getting more fit every day. The components of high vibratory rate consist of energy, enthusiasm, confidence, belief and clarity. Fit people maximize each component and the result is a mindset of sustained concentration on their desired outcome. The high rate of vibration keeps motivation high and temptation low, and it's accessible to anyone. So while fat people are losing energy, fit people are gaining it.

Fat Loser Quote

66 *Energy is life. Without it, you have nothing. Being fat consumes massive amounts of physical, mental, and emotional energy faster than anything else. Fat sucks the life out of your days while it slowly kills you. Get rid of it and you're energy level will skyrocket! You'll feel great and look even better. You are one simple decision away from boundless energy and enthusiasm. The clock is ticking. What are waiting for?* 99

Critical Thinking Question

Can you imagine having 20, 30, or even 50 percent more physical, mental, and spiritual energy in your life?

Action Step

Begin to notice the increase in energy as you move from success to success in the weight loss/fitness process. Just making a decision to get fit and the good thoughts and feelings it creates will give you a major energy boost.

Fat people berate themselves when they don't see immediate results

Fit people reward themselves for execution

The middle-class mindset that plaques fat people expects instant results. When it doesn't happen, fat people get down on themselves and wonder why they even started the process. Fit people know results take time, and they reward themselves for sticking to their program even when their results aren't favorable. Since their commitment is long term, short term results are of little concern. World-class thinking drives their behavior and guides them to build eating and exercise habits that serve their best interests. Since fat people often make weak commitments to change, they need daily reinforcement just to stick to their diet. When they don't experience immediate success, they often revert back to their old habits, which destroy what little self-confidence they have. So while fat people are their own worst enemies, fit people are their own best friends. One of their secrets is execution based goal setting, which focuses on executing the actions you can control in place of results. Results aren't ignored; they're simply monitored as opposed to being focused on. This puts the performer in complete control of their success, and keeps them on the road to fitness. The fact is, sometimes weight loss is fast, and other times it's slow. If you're emotionally addicted to quick results, that habit must be broken. Getting fit is a life-long proposition. Getting to your ideal weight is only the beginning of the process. The key is getting physically fit and staying physically fit for life. That's why developing new eating and exercise habits are the secret to success. This is why fit people reward themselves for execution. They know once their new habits are built, the struggle to lose and maintain weight will gently fade away.

Fat Loser Quote

❝ *The great ones know the execution of a well designed strategy will always lead to success. This is why they reward themselves for execution whether they're getting results or not. They've learned that timelines are hard to predict yet success is inevitable if they stay the course and execute the plan. The masses must see instant results, yet often time changes don't happen immediately in diet and exercise. The body might be holding onto excess weight as a security measure, only to release it as necessary. Results might be the only thing that counts, but they are the last part of a multifaceted process. Reward yourself for execution, knowing that eventually the results will follow.* ❞

Critical Thinking Question

Are you rewarding yourself for sticking to your diet and exercise program on a daily, weekly and monthly basis? Will your rewards have more impact during the habit change process or after the struggle is over?

Action Step

Just for today, give yourself a small (non-food) reward for being 100% compliant on your diet and exercise program, and notice how it affects you. If it works, implement new rewards every day or at least once a week. Once the struggle is over and your new habits are in place, you won't need rewards. You'll feel so good physically and mentally you'll wonder why you didn't get fit sooner.

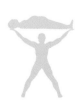

Fat people want to be recognized for suffering

Fit people want to be recognized for success

Fat people who haven't fully committed to a healthy diet and exercise program thrive on sympathy from others. After years of failing on diets, many have become emotionally addicted to people feeling sorry for them. Anytime they're out to dinner they're sure to let everyone know they're adhering to their diet and suffering. This not only rewards them emotionally, it also prepares them for eventual failure. Surely their friends and family will understand that no human being could succeed long term through all that suffering? Each time they fail, they're showered with more sympathy. This endless loop of emotional addiction to sympathy is one of the most debilitating mindsets of the middle class. It's passed down from generation to generation, until a maverick in the family breaks the cycle. Fit people don't get thin and healthy for anyone but themselves. They succeed because they believe they're worth it. Fit people who get fat don't stay fat for long because they have learned to think fit. A fit person in a fat body never feels comfortable. When they look in the mirror and see mediocrity it feels out of place. They have a healthy self-image and seeing a fat, bloated, distorted body reflected back at them makes them feel as though they're living in someone else's skin. This cognitive incongruity drives them to make immediate changes in their diet and exercise program until they are fit and healthy again. People can applaud them, express sympathy, and even attempt to dissuade them, but nothing stops them. They move forward like a locomotive driven by passion and emotion until they look in the mirror and see themselves again. The fit person's reward comes from within, and they are willing to forgo the pleasure-based rewards of the present for the gratification of the future.

Fat Loser Quote

❝ *Everyone loves recognition, including the world class. The difference in thinking is the great ones don't need to be recognized for the sacrifices and suffering along the road to success. They just want to be recognized for the success itself. The masses crave instant gratification and want sympathy for their struggle. This is a trap that derails many people when they fail to find the outpouring of sympathy they require to continue. Millions of people start diets every day, and most fail. Expect to get your recognition when you've earned it, and not a day before. This mindset will keep you focused on succeeding instead of suffering.* ❞

Critical Thinking Question

Are you searching for sympathy for your temporary suffering or looking forward to a lifetime of recognition for your fitness success?

Action Step

Invest thirty seconds today in imagining how your friends and family will respond to your fitness success. Think about how you will be treated with more respect. Flash a picture in your mind of how others will look at you when you walk into a room. Ponder how you will become an inspiration to others who are struggling with their weight.

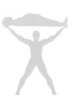

Fat people are products of middle-class programming

Fit people are products world-class programming

F at people aren't fat because they're less educated or intelligent than fit people. They're fat because they've bought into the middle-class programming of the masses. People of influence during childhood and adolescence start the process, and the media, advertisers, friends and co-workers solidify it. Even some well known psychologists and other influential mental health professionals are publically advising fat people to accept their fate and stop berating themselves. In essence, they're being told to give up because they're not tough enough to get fit. This is middle-class thinking at its worst. Mental health professionals have been advising people for years not to have too high of an expectation for their lives, lest they be disappointed and end up unhappy. They imply that most of us aren't mentally tough enough to fight for what we want and persist until we get it, so we shouldn't expect too much and simply be glad we have a roof over our head and clothes on our backs. These so called experts aren't espousing this nonsense out of malice; they're suggesting it because they believe it's the right thing to do. In America, the land of limitless opportunity, more people have held themselves back through middle-class thinking than anything else. Luckily the founding fathers were world-class thinkers, or we'd still be drinking tea in the afternoon! Fit people categorically reject middle-class thinking and embrace the mindset of the great ones. Not only do they have a crystal clear vision of their ultimate physique, they expect to see it in the mirror. They listen to the language of the world class, and immerse their consciousness in empowering thoughts and inspirational philosophies. The idea of accepting themselves as fat is ludicrous and laughable, and anyone suggesting such pseudo-wisdom won't be around them for long.

Fat Loser Quote

❝ The average person speaks at a rate of 150-200 words per minute. The average persons self-talk is about 1300 words per minute. This one piece of information has the power to make or break you in the weight loss control process, because it tells us that the real power of programming lies in the way we talk to ourselves all day long. Our self-talk is a significant agent of change we can all employ. ❞

Critical Thinking Question

Are you ready to let go of the middle-class programming that allowed you to get fat, and accept full responsibility for all of your future results?

Action Step

Start listening to world-class beliefs and philosophies every day until they are programmed into your conscious and sub-conscious minds. Invest in a CD album called The Making of a Million Dollar Mind at www.milliondollarmind.com

Fat people believe they know how to get fit

Fit people are learning machines

F at people have usually lost and gained dozens if not hundreds of pounds throughout their lifetime, which leads them to believe they know everything there is to know about this subject. The truth is their knowledge is limited to short term success and long term failure. If fat people knew how to be thin and healthy long term, they'd be fit. This is another example of self-delusion clouding objective judgment, and it's easy to fall into. Fit people are always searching for answers, and are open minded to new ideas, systems, and philosophies that will help them get healthier. In the age of rapidly advancing scientific discovery, more efficient and effective methods of getting fit are being discovered every day. Whether it's raising their level of awareness in common everyday dieting and exercise wisdom, or studying the latest trends, fit people approach learning process with a beginner's mind and an open heart. While fat people are embarrassed to ask for help, fit people hire personal coaches, trainers and mentors to help them succeed. They are able to bypass their egos and operate from a spirit-based consciousness, which is another mental toughness secret of the world class. This mindset allows them to become learning machines and acquire wisdom from anyone with expertise. Since fat people are hindered by an ego-based mindset that knows it all, they miss new strategies that could help them get fit. Meanwhile, fit people stay open minded and continue to become more educated. This is one the reasons the fat get fatter and the fit, fitter.

Fat Loser Quote

❝ World-class thinkers are like human sponges. They soak up specialized knowledge and ancient wisdom like the masses soak up television and video games. New diet discoveries and formulations are presented on a regular basis, and fit people are in the habit of searching for and finding the latest and greatest ways of getting healthier every day. Fit people are also up to date on the latest trends in exercise science, always looking to increase their efficiency and effectiveness. While the middle class is convinced they know everything they need to know, the great ones stay on the cutting edge of every area of life they care about improving. ❞

Critical Thinking Question

Are you tapping into the expertise of others who can make your fitness journey easier and more enjoyable?

Action Step

Study as many world-class experts on health and fitness as you can. Beginning today, invest 15 minutes studying an expert you respect.

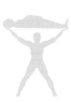

Fat people believe the emotional responses that made them fat will make them thin

Fit people change their emotional responses to alter their results

Habitual emotional responses have the power to create massive success or colossal failure. Most of these responses are acquired in childhood and retained for life. For example, when fat people hear the word diet the most common emotional response is frustration and anger. When fit people hear the word diet, they picture their body being even healthier, and they experience the emotion of excitement. When fat people hear the word exercise, they feel psychological pressure and loathing of an activity they don't like. Some fat people despise exercise in any form, and hate is the emotion they experience. Through years of conditioning, all of us have developed habitual emotional responses that either help or hurt us. Fat people who don't change their emotional responses to eating and exercise will fail to get and stay fit. Since fat people are in the habit of eating to alter their emotions, changing their emotional responses is critical to their success. Fit people know the powerful role emotions play with all human beings, and that we are primarily emotional creatures. All negative emotional responses to any positive activity, idea or philosophy that leads to greater fitness must be systematically eliminated to insure long term success. These harmful responses must be erased and replaced with new, empowering responses that move you toward your fitness goals. Like anything of a habitual nature, emotional responses can be drastically altered in less than 30 days through persistent practice. After the changes are made fit people simply guard the door of their consciousness to make sure the old habits don't get back in. This guarding process gets easier and easier as the new habits become more ingrained daily.

Fat Loser Quote

❝ Mental toughness is about emotional control. If you want to get fit, you must adopt the emotional responses of a fit person. When a fit person feels hunger, she thinks 'opportunity'. When she feels too tired to exercise, she thinks 'If I were in better shape, I wouldn't be tired'. When she thinks about cheating on her diet, she thinks 'It's way too slippery of a slope to risk". Emotional responses are upgraded one event at a time, one day at a time. It's a tedious process in the beginning, but once you have the ball rolling, momentum takes over and speeds the change. ❞

Critical Thinking Question

Are you using your old emotional responses that made you fat or creating new ones that will make you fit?

Action Step

Start a new emotional response today to the word 'diet'. From now on this word excites you, because it's the path to a life of world- class health, energy, abundance and fitness.

Fat people think they have forever to change

Fit people have a sense of urgency

Fat people are always postponing getting fit for some perfect time in the future. Self-delusion tells them their health is not at risk and they have the rest of their lives to change. The truth is, being fat is like having a ticking time bomb on your body without a time clock. This is especially scary for the morbidly obese, who are 'whistling past the graveyard'. With their thinking grounded in objective reality, fit people have a sense of urgency about getting thin and healthy. Their mindset is to take action while they still have a choice. Good health can deteriorate quickly, and tempting fate is a gamble fit people aren't willing to take. This sense of urgency is a critical component of world-class thinking, and fit people carry it into every aspect of their lives. Like many of the mental toughness secrets of the world class, sense of urgency is both a philosophy and a habit of thought. The middle class is famous for procrastination, especially when it comes to areas of life that are uncomfortable. If I've learned anything about people in the last 24 years of study, it's that the downfall of the average person is an overwhelming desire to be comfortable. In the mindset of the masses, comfort is king. While the great ones are doing whatever it takes to succeed, the majority of the population is just trying to avoid pain. The sad truth is many people come to the end of their lives with feelings of regret for not taking more risks and going after their dreams. It's difficult to maximize your potential when your primary focus is playing it safe. It's no different with fitness. Fat people suffer the negative effects of obesity every day, but they somehow believe it's easier than sticking to a healthy diet and exercise program. Fit people are baffled by this lopsided trade-off, but it makes perfect sense to someone clouded by delusion. The solution is simple: stop promising yourself you're going to get fit someday, and do it now! The clock is ticking. What are you waiting for?

Fat Loser Quote

❝ When you find yourself about to cheat, ask yourself this question: if you don't stick to your diet now, then when? Next time? The time after that? All of us are on borrowed time, and when we're done, we're done. There is no second chance. The time to act is now. This problem must be solved, and it won't go away on its own. As a matter of fact, it's going to get harder every time you fail. Why not just solve it once and for all and move on with your life? ❞

Critical Thinking Question

Do you have a sense of urgency about getting fit, or are you tempting fate by deluding yourself into believing you have forever?

Action Step

Decide to get fit now instead of later. Not next week, not after the holidays or next summer. Do it now, while there's still time. Do it now, while you still have a choice.

Fat people believe fitness is complicated

Fit people believe fitness is simple

Fat people are often intimidated by the complexities of the weight loss/maintenance process. Fit people leave the complex configuring of calories and their counterparts to the doctors and scientists who create the diets. Fit people focus on their part of the equation: sticking to the diet. Fat people are always searching for the perfect diet instead of finding a diet they can stick to. There is no perfect diet. If you're going to get thin and healthy, you are going to pay a price. But you're paying a price right now for being fat, aren't you? The fact is, a price will be paid one way or another, so why not choose the one that offers the most benefits? There are no benefits to being fat, except you can eat like a pig without restrictions. The problem is, if you eat like a pig, you probably look like a pig. Unless you've got the metabolism of a racehorse, unrestricted eating will eventually lead to disease and death. This is one of the reasons fit people see getting fit as a simple decision, followed by a short period of heavy discipline that eventually leads to a light discipline for life. Getting fit is the only intelligent choice. It's either get fit or suffer the physical, psychological, and social consequences for the rest of your short life. Making simple facts complex is a symptom of middle-class thinking. The masses love to play the victim, so they often exaggerate the complexity and sacrifice of something as simple as getting fit. World-class thinkers are just the opposite. They keep the simple, simple, and are masters of making the complex, simple. This removes the intimidation factor from the task they're attempting, and gives them the belief they need to conquer things the masses run away from. So remember that getting fit is a simple decision followed by simple discipline. Nothing more, nothing less. You can do it!

Fat Loser Quote

“ *Technology is making exercise simpler and more fun every day, and the closer you get to your ideal weight, the more you will enjoy it. Exercise leaves fat people gasping for air. Exercise gives fit people more energy than when they started. Getting fit builds two of the life's most important habits: regular exercise and good eating habits. Your success in these two areas will give you the confidence to build a life most people only dream of.* **”**

Critical Thinking Question

Are you making fitness more complicated than it needs to be?

Action Step

**Break your exercise down into simple, manageable parts.
Keep your workouts short and focused.
Don't waste time talking and socializing.
Get to the gym and get it done.**

Fat people have middle-class self-talk

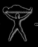

Fit people have world-class self-talk

Fat people talk themselves out of being thin. They tell themselves that someday they'll lose weight and get thin and healthy, but they that day never comes. They tell themselves they deserve to eat whatever they want whenever they want because they're depressed, stressed, or bored. They tell themselves it will be more painful not eating their favorite foods than it is being fat. Is it any mystery why the fat get fatter? Fit people also talk to themselves. Fit people tell themselves a thin, healthy and attractive body feels better than any food will ever taste. They tell themselves they feel better and have more energy eating healthy foods. They tell themselves exercise is fun and it feels fantastic knowing you're getting stronger and healthier every day. Is it any mystery the fit get fitter? The language we use with ourselves is the most powerful of all the mental conditioning tools. Human beings are in a constant conversation with themselves, including in our dreams when we sleep. Nothing has more power to change our beliefs and behaviors than positive self- talk. It's the most underrated self-empowerment strategy in the history of performance psychology. Fat people develop their self-talk scripts from the masses, and much of it is integrated and executed unconsciously. Fit people develop their self-talk scripts from world-class performers, and most of it is integrated and executed with acute awareness. The difference is fit people know the power of positive, strategically directed self-talk; and fat people don't. The masses don't even discuss strategies like self-talk, nor are they taught in schools. The result of this ignorance is a population of people programming their minds with the random self-talk of the mediocre masses. This is not for you. Decide today what messages of hope, inspiration and encouragement you should be reciting to yourself on a daily basis. If you're thinking this is hokey, that's middle-class thinking coming through. Reject the messages of the masses and get mentally tough with yourself by conditioning your mind for fitness.

Fat Loser Quote

Champions know that everything affects everything. That's why you'll hear fit people speaking only the language of love, abundance and gratitude. Every little success, no matter how small, has a domino effect. Getting fit will positively impact every area of your life. This law also applies to failure. The little piece of candy you eat might not seem like a big deal, but the ripple effect of this simple act of non-compliance has the power to unravel months of habit formation. The one fear-based conversation you have with someone may seem unimportant, but its impact on your state of mind is substantial. The law doesn't care if you use it to help or hurt you. Nature is neutral. Decide today to contemplate the consequences of all of your actions every day, no matter how meaningless they appear.

Action Step

Start upgrading your self-talk today by
focusing on the world-class language of
love, abundance, gratitude and optimism.
Your self-talk will have a dramatic impact
on your belief system, and will drive your
behavior to support your upgraded beliefs.

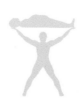

Fat people rely on diets, pills and potions

Fit people rely on themselves

Fat people are waiting for the next latest/greatest diet that's going to save them from themselves. They believe they're fat because fast food chains are on every corner, restaurants are serving giant portions, and food manufacturers are injecting chemicals that create addictions to unhealthy foods. They blame everything and everyone but themselves, and when they do accept responsibility, they go into a depression from thinking about how unworthy and weak they are. If this is you get over it! Almost everyone in the population has gotten fat during some period of their life. Getting fat doesn't make you weak, it makes you human. So you got fat, so what? Join the club. If I hadn't gained forty pounds of fat five years ago you wouldn't be reading this book. I know how you feel and so do most people. You're not alone, and you deserve to be thin and healthy. Fit people screw up, too, but they take responsibility and then go to work to solve the problem. Don't waste time wallowing in self-pity, and you can't afford to feed the habit of searching for sympathy. Not only will playing the victim keep you fat, it will also hold you back in every other area of your life. The masses love to commiserate, sharing stories of hardship for the emotional reward of being in the same boat as everyone else. The boat the majority of the population is in is called the USS Middle Class, and you should avoid boarding it under any circumstances. Seeking sympathy in moderation wouldn't be so harmful if it weren't so addictive and habitual, but it is. Seeking sympathy is the crack cocaine of the masses, and once you have that monkey on your back, it's difficult to get rid of it. Choose self-reliance instead. Grow up and stop making excuses for being fat. I mean, really: is a life of mediocrity that appealing? Don't wait to be great. Go for it now, while you still have a choice.

Fat Loser Quote

66 *Anytime a world-class thinker embarks on a big project, he knows he'll have to rely mostly on himself to make it happen. Mentor and support teams are great, but in the end success is in the hands of the performer. The more successes you experience, the more self-reliant you become. While the masses are waiting for the hero on the white horse to save them, the great ones are realize no one is coming to the rescue.* 99

Critical Thinking Question

Are you self-reliant, or are you waiting for a hero on a white horse to save you from yourself?

Action Step

Accept the fact that no one is coming to the rescue, and your level of fitness depends completely on you.

Fat people don't connect fitness with sexual energy

Fit people know sexual energy increases through fitness

People who've made the transition from fat to fit have a secret few are willing to share, and that's the impact getting in shape has on their level of sexual energy. This massive increase occurs physically, mentally, and spiritually. It's no surprise that looking good makes you feel good, and this winning combination makes you more attractive to others. The middle-class mindset, rooted in fear and scarcity, rarely acknowledges this fact due to the mental and emotional baggage they've been programmed with about sex since childhood. World-class thinkers embrace this beautiful and exciting facet of human existence, and they embrace the idea of increased interest and pleasure. The benefits of increased sexual energy go beyond the obvious, because like any raw form of energy, it can be converted and focused in any direction you choose. Athletes have used this technique for years, and so have many other ambitious performers looking for an edge. Sexual energy is like a shot of adrenaline that heightens your awareness and keeps you focused. Think about the physical, mental and emotional intensity that occurs before a sexual encounter and imagine harnessing it to be directed toward a business or personal goal. Fit people who use weight training also experience heightened levels of sexual energy and are able to use it to increase their strength and stamina. Being fat has the opposite effect, which is one of the reasons so many couples experience problems in their sex lives. If you're fat and disgusted with yourself every time you look in the mirror, the last thing on your mind is sex. And if both partners are fat, the problem is compounded. I mean, really: who wants to have sex when they can barely handle seeing themselves naked? Since the media sells advertising to companies patronized primarily by the middle class, you won't hear much about this phenomenon. That doesn't mean it doesn't exist. Just know this is yet another benefit that awaits you when you join the ranks of the fit.

Fat Loser Quote

❝ Getting fit will reignite your sex life like nothing else. There's nothing like getting in tune with your body. Your increased energy, vitality and self-esteem will positively impact your love life on every level. ❞

Critical Thinking Question

How much pleasure are you sacrificing in your sex life because you're fat?

Action Step

Let go of the delusion that being fat isn't hurting your sex life. Fat is a major turn-off, and being fat reduces your sex drive and inhibits your performance.

Fat people lack hope

Fit people are excited about their future

It's hard to have hope about looking and feeling better when you're getting fatter every day. Fat people are out of control and they know it, yet feel powerless to change. Being fat creates a downward spiral of negative effects that drain the hope and optimism out of the most enthusiastic people. There's not one single advantage to being fat, and the downsides can be deadly, yet millions of people choose obesity every day. Being fat doesn't just happen; it's a choice you make with every meal. It's something we do to ourselves, yet are quick to blame others. Fit people look forward to a future where they will be healthier and fitter. Fit people are in control of their minds and bodies, and that gives them a level of confidence fat people can't imagine. The thought is; if I can control my mind and body, I can do anything I set my sights on! This belief becomes a self-fulfilling prophecy that gets stronger every day with each success. Eventually the fit person believes anything is possible, and the world is at his/her feet. After several months of going from fat to fit these benefits are so numerous that a fit person no longer has to exercise much discipline. If fat people could only get a glimpse of life as a fit person they wouldn't ever go back to being fat. The critical thinking question is this: Is it more difficult to change your eating and exercise habits than it is to wake up every day with no hope? Before answering, be sure to consider that the heart of the behavior change process is only 21-30 days in duration. For some people those first few weeks are easy, for others it's tough. After that, the level of discipline and willpower required decreases every day until it's something you have to remind yourself to be conscious of. It doesn't mean you won't be ever be tempted by doughnuts and ice cream, they simply won't have the power they once had, which makes it easier to walk away. Now do you see why fit people are excited about the future?

Fat Loser Quote

66 *Fit people know their future is going to be better than their past because they are getting healthier every day. Fitness increases feelings of hope, optimism and enthusiasm for life. It's the centerpiece on the table of the future. While fat people are getting fatter and more depressed every day, fit people are reaping the rewards of their organized discipline. One group knows today is as good as it gets, and the other knows today is just the beginning of a brilliant future.* 99

Critical Thinking Question
Have you carefully crafted your
vision of your future as a fit person?

Action Step
Once your vision is written, read it every
morning and ingrain the images of the future
into your consciousness. This will help keep
you on track when the going gets tough.

Fat people give up on themselves

Fit people never say die

Most fat people have attempted to get fit, but either succeeded and gained the weight back or failed and gave up. The cost in health and quality of life is substantial, but the cost in self-confidence is devastating. If failing to get fit was just about physical health, it would be harmful enough, but the mental, emotional and spiritual effects make it too high a price to pay. That's why failure is not an option. Fit people are acutely aware of what's at stake when it comes to getting and staying fit. That's why they have been widely criticized as 'health nuts' and 'gym freaks'. Being thin and healthy is a good enough reason to fight the good fight, but it turns out that this is just the tip of the iceberg. That's why fit people do whatever it takes to succeed and never say die. When most people are tired, emotionally worn out and ready to quit, fit people are just warming up. Fat people go into this fight expecting a gentle transition. Fit people go into this expecting a fight. When they wake up in the morning dying to eat something unhealthy they're not surprised. When they go to bed at night with their stomach growling they're ready for it. Fit people expect to pay a price for success. They know nothing good comes easily, and they commit to doing whatever it takes with their eyes wide open. When family, friends and co-workers pressure them to stray from their diet; they're mentally prepared for it. Nothing takes them by surprise so they rarely go off course. A key component of their success is knowing the battle of the bulge is a battle most people lose. This makes them prepare to persevere through the pain. So the real question is not "can you get fit"? The real question is, "are you willing to never say die until you get fit?"

Critical Thinking Question

Have you finally come to the realization that getting fit is a war that must be won? Do you really believe failure is an option?

Action Step

Decide you will do whatever it takes to get fit and that you will never say die. This isn't a game. If you fail, you will continue to get fatter and sicker, and you will eventually die fat. The only thing separating you from a life of disease and a life of abundant health is a rock solid decision. Make it today and watch your energy soar!

Fat people refuse to suffer

Fit people know why they must suffer

The most unpopular word in the history of the Mental Toughness Institute for Weight Control (aka The Fat Losers Program) is 'suffer'. The critical thinking question we ask people to ask themselves is 'why must I suffer?' The premise of the question is grounded in the objective reality which says changing habitual behavior involves some level of suffering. The positive thinking purists hate this question because it predisposes that suffering must take place. They've been conditioned to believe if they ignore reality it will go away, which is the primary reason many of these people fail to get fit. If positive thinking was all it took to succeed, they wouldn't be fat in the first place. The problem with delusional thinking in this context is the softening of the language often precedes the softening of the person's resolve. When you go into a fight expecting a picnic, you fold up your basket and blanket at the first sign of ants. When you go into a fight fully prepared to suffer you're not surprised when it gets tough. Here's a shot of objective reality: if it were so easy to get fit everyone would be fit. If it were so easy to get rich everyone would be rich. I could recite an entire laundry list that the positive thinking purists say are easy while most are failing. Fit people look for the positive but prepare for the negative. While positive thinkers love to debate the semantics of language, critical thinkers just shut up and do the work. Whether you believe you will suffer or not doesn't make any difference. Whether you are prepared to suffer or not makes all the difference. If you're under the impression you can think your way into getting fit, think again. World-class thinking is a great start, but free will is the bottom line when it comes to succeeding. You can be as positive or negative as you want, but sticking to your diet and exercise program is the only thing that will make you thin and healthy.

Fat Loser Quote

❝ *Become an observer of your own habit patterns, because they are the treasure map to your results. Most people have middle-class habit patterns, which is why they get middle-class results. Getting hung up on semantics and meaningless details is a common habit of the middle class. The masses are famous for wasting an inordinate amount of mental energy contemplating and fighting for details that don't move them closer to their goals. Upgrade your habits and the results will follow. All of your results come directly from your dominant habit patterns.* ❞

Critical Thinking Question

As an intelligent and educated person, do you honestly believe you're going to go from fat to fit without suffering?

Action Step

Mentally prepare yourself to experience a light to moderate level of physical, psychological, and emotional suffering. The pain isn't extreme and won't last long, but it's serious enough to make most people quit. That's why you need to prepare yourself before it begins. Remember that any time you make a major habit change you will pay a price. Prepare now so you won't be surprised when the going gets tough.

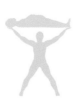

Fat people ignore fit people

Fit people follow role models

I'll go to my grave never understanding why fat people don't find out what fit people do and copy it. Not that it's any different in any other area where people are failing. When I was broke, I interviewed people who were rich. I knew there had to be something they were doing that I wasn't, or even a series of things. That turned out to be true, and their advice to me was to change my habits and copy theirs. Was it easy? No. Did my old habits die hard? Yes. It was the toughest thing I've ever done. I had the self-doubt, naysayers and late nights of wondering if I was wasting my time mimicking millionaires. They told me to expect a fight because old habits, especially habits of thought, are deeply ingrained in your consciousness, and it takes mental toughness and persistence to erase and replace them. It turned out to be the same mental toughness I coached great athletes on. Now it was time to see if I could use that same strength to build a fortune. Of course these people were right, and my old habits eventually gave up and new habits took over. (Most of them, anyway.) These rich people taught me when I thought the way they thought and did the things they did, money would flow like water. They were right, and it changed my life. So did I succeed because I'm so smart? No. I'm an ordinary person of average intelligence. I won't be in the running for a Nobel Prize or curing cancer anytime soon. The secret of my success, and the success of people far more successful than me, is finding out what other successful people do and copying it. That's about as simple and linear as it gets. The problem is nobody does it. Or more accurately, a very small percentage of the population does it. Probably the same one percent that owns the majority of the wealth. This book is the result of my getting fat and asking fit people how to fix it. Then I copied their physical, mental and emotional habits and got fit. Then I created the Fat Loser Program and wrote this book to save you the time of having to do all the research. All you have to do is 'follow the yellow brick road.' Are you ready?

Are you ready?

Fat Loser Quote

❝ Fat people pay no attention to how fat their closest family and friends are. They're largely unaware of the disastrous effects other fat people are having on their thinking. Fit people know hanging out with other fit people is critical to their ongoing success and fit-consciousness development. Fit people don't associate with other fit people because they believe they're better, they associate with them because they believe they are better at staying fit and they want to grow from their exposure. While the middle class sees this strategic association as elitism, the great ones see it as a practical and powerful strategy. ❞

Critical Thinking Question

Do you have a fit friend or mentor you can use as a role model?

Action Step

Identify someone who exemplifies the level of fitness you wish to attain, and ask him/her to serve as your role model.

Fat people don't know why they're fat

Fit people know exactly why they are fit

Fat people get on the scale and are stunned when they continue gaining weight. I know, because I did the same thing. Self-delusion seems simple but can be very tricky. It had me saying things like, "but I only had one bag of chips, how could I gain two pounds?" Broke people don't like to budget their money and fat people don't like to budget their food. They like to eat whatever they want, whenever they want, in any combination they want, yet they expect to be thin and healthy. Like people failing in any area of life, they keep repeating the same behaviors and habits while expecting different results. Fat people often believe they deserve to lose weight because they're cutting back or exercising more. This is a recipe for frustration and failure. It's like driving in a circle around Miami while expecting to end up in Atlanta. While fat people are sometimes willing to do the work, they're not committed enough to formulate a plan and follow it to the letter. This is their emotional hedge that lets them off the hook in case they fail, which is imminent. Then they blame the diet for not working. This is why 99% percent compliance to your diet and exercise program is not enough. You don't go into a war and say you're going to give it 99%. America learned that lesson in Vietnam. We called it a "Military Action" and the Vietnamese called it a war. They were 100% committed and they won a war that was all but impossible for them to win. That's the difference the extra 1% makes. Fit people know why they are fit because there are consciously aware of everything that goes into their mouths. They know exactly how much they exercise and leave nothing to chance. How about you? Are you asleep or awake?

Fat Loser Quote

" Fit people know exactly what they did to get fit. They are conscious of everything they eat and every form of exercise they participate in. Fat people pack on 50 pounds unconsciously, have no idea how it happened, and swear it's only 20 pounds. This phenomenon is no different in any other area of life. Broke people have no idea why they're broke, yet rich people know exactly how they got rich. People with broken relationships are shocked when they're served with divorce papers, while people with great marriages are very aware of why they are so successful. Unhappy people are always searching for the cause of their distress, while happy people have a formula that works for them over and over.

Awareness and attention to detail has always been a hallmark of the most successful people in the world. "

Critical Thinking Question

Do you know why you allowed yourself to get fat? Do you know why you're getting fit?

Action Step

Do some soul searching today and identify the physical and emotional reasons you allowed yourself to get fat. Next, identify the physical and emotional motivators that are driving you to get fit. The more clearly you can track your behavior of the past, the more clearly you can chart your course for the future.

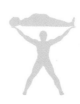

Fat people believe they have to succeed on their own

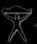

Fit people build a mentor and support team

One of the hallmarks of middle-class thinking is the belief you have to do everything on your own. We're programmed as children to be self-reliant to survive, which is good, but not in every application. Why not move from linear to non linear thinking and leverage the intelligence, experience and know-how of others? Why not build a team to help you get thin and healthy? The reason is another downfall of the middle-class mindset: ego. Our egos get in the way of doing things in our own best interest. The masses are programmed to believe if you ask for help it makes you less than the person you're asking. Objective reality tells us that everyone has specific talents and blind spots. Logic tells us to maximize our talents and minimize our blinds spots by tapping into the talents of others. That's why fit people build a mentor team to guide them and a support team to help them emotionally when things get tough. World-class thinkers transcend the ego-based thinking of the masses and tap into their spirit. The religious call it God and the secular say consciousness, but whatever label you assign it the result is the same. The spirit based mindset welcomes all the help and support it can get. That's why so many fit people hire personal trainers and coaches. They don't need to succeed on their own, they just want to win. When they need help they ask for it without guilt or shame. Their spirit based consciousness allows them to stay open to more efficient ways of getting fit, as well as strategies to reduce the suffering that often goes along with any major habit change. So do you have your mentor/support team in place, or is your ego keeping you from asking for help? Is it more important to satisfy an insatiable ego or get fit?

Fat Loser Quote

❝ *Fit people prepare to win the weight loss war by building mentor and support teams. The mentor team serves as their guide to eating and exercise. The support team serves as their emotional support system in times of stress, disappointment, or any other problem that threatens to knock the champion off track. As strong and self-reliant as the great ones are, they know they are still fallible human beings subject to the same emotional storms as everyone else. These two teams are the performer's insurance policy to achieving any goal or dream they set their sights on.* ❞

Critical Thinking Question

Have you built a mentor and support
team to help guide and inspire you
on your journey to fitness?

Action Step

Start today to assemble your mentor and
support team, and tap into each of them as
needed. They will serve as your insurance
policy in your quest for fitness.

Fat people allow others to knock them off track

Fit people know how to say no

The masses have always been, and will always be heavily influenced by the thoughts and opinions of others. The negative effect of peer pressure on the middle class extends beyond adolescence into adulthood. Fat people on a diet are often derailed at the urging of friends, family and co-workers who pressure them to abandon their diet for a variety of reasons. With little confidence in themselves and a poor track record to run on, fat people attempting to get fit often fall prey to the mindset of the masses. Fit people listen to their mentor and support teams and cocoon themselves during the early stages of habit alteration, knowing this 3-4 week period is the most critical time in the process. Fit people know the importance of blocking out negative influences and learning to ignore the opinions of the middle class. Their greatest test occurs on weekends, holidays, and other special occasions where well-intending family and friends apply massive doses of emotional pressure to break their diet. While most people believe cheating on one meal is no big deal, fit people are aware of the dire consequences of severing the newly sown thread of a new habit and the domino effect that occurs as a result. One meal turns into a full day, which turns into "I'll start back on Monday". That's why fit people get comfortable saying no to even the slightest compromise in their diet. They know that every time they reject someone pressuring them to cheat, they get stronger and more committed. Fit people realize the battle for optimum health is a battle that must be won if they're going to get the most out of life, and they refuse to allow some well- meaning but potentially harmful middle-class thinker to push them off track. The question every fat person must ask themselves is: am I willing to stand up for myself and stick to the diet, or give someone else the power to reinforce my old losing habits?

Fat Loser Quote

66 *Fit people have learned how to say no to themselves and others. All they see is the goal, and everything else must give way. Saying no to unhealthy foods and the people who coerce them into eating these foods is the heart of this habit. Saying no to old habits of thought is another. While fat people are worried about disappointing other people by saying no, fit people are more concerned with missing the goal and disappointing themselves. Learning to say no to things that don't serve your best interests is a habit you must build in order to achieve any major success.* 99

Critical Thinking Question

Have you learned how to say no to people who may unknowingly try to knock you off track? Have you learned how to say no to yourself?

Action Step

Make a decision to distance yourself from people who refuse to support you in your fitness goals. Your life is at stake, and this calls for drastic measures. Just say no to spending time with people unless they are in harmony with your biggest goals and dreams.

Fat people are addicted to food

Fit people are addicted to success

Fat people are addicted to how foods make them feel the same way a drunk gets addicted to booze. The drunk blames the liquor companies and the fat person blames the food manufacturers, restaurants and anything/anyone else they can. The word addiction is often used loosely in reference to food, but it appeals to the middle class because it absolves them from taking responsibility for their behavior. Eating creates instant, short term pleasure, and pleasure is the most popular mood choice known to man. But the fact is it's still a choice. No one comes over to your house and shoves doughnuts and cookies down your throat. Fat people have no one to blame but themselves, yet the word addiction implies they are genetically predisposed to be obese and powerless over food. Again, the middle-class mindset always looks to be the victim and escape responsibility. Fit people make a valiant effort to become addicted to a healthy diet and robust exercise program that serve their best interests. Like the fat person gaining pleasure from food, fit people experience instant gratification from the endorphin rush of exercise. The bonus is they also experience the positive feelings generated from sticking to their goal and the subsequent boost in self-confidence that accompanies it. Some people call this a 'healthy addiction', but the fact is, the individual is always in control. No matter how much pull unhealthy foods have, you will always have free will to make the healthy choice. Don't let the establishment convince you that you are powerless over food because they've given you a way out of taking responsibility by labeling your poor eating habits as an addiction. Grow up and take control of your food choices and reject the pop psychology that sells the masses on the idea they are powerless.

It's a lie that will keep you fat forever.

Fat Loser Quote

66 *Well-meaning family, friends, and even health care professionals will try to convince you to just be happy being fat, and learn to accept your failure in this area. They'll tell you if you don't expect much you won't be disappointed. The masses have always been focused on how to avoid pain, while the classes are focused on manifesting their dreams. Disappointment and failure are part of life. Get tough and persist until you succeed! Go for what you want while there's still time. The clock is ticking.* 99

Critical Thinking Question

What do you place more value on in your life: food or success?

Action Step

Start telling yourself food is only important for creating energy and sustaining life. Stop telling yourself how much you love food. The food you claim to love so much is making you miserable and doesn't care if it kills you.

Fat people are influenced by fat people

Fit people have become desensitized to the opinions of fat people

Fat people love to commiserate with other fat people who reinforce the idea that fat is OK, not dangerous to your health, and the direct result of an uncontrollable outside force. Fat people hang around fat people. Broke people hang around broke people. Fit people hang around fit people. While fit people are getting inspired and motivated associating with other fit people, fat people are slipping deeper into the cesspool of mediocrity through ongoing exposure to the consciousness that made them fat. The winners in American society have often been labeled as elitists for their unwillingness to allow the average person into their inner circle. As someone who has interviewed these people for 24 years, I can say with some authority that their behavior has little to do with elitism and everything to do with calculated strategy. You see, most winners come from humble beginnings, and they have a burning desire to hold on to their new success. Fit people, just like any other group that is winning, know the power associations have on their thinking. Many of them are recovering middle-class thinkers who can't afford to be exposed to the thought viruses of the masses for fear they will revert to their old habits of thought. Just like a recovering alcoholic avoiding a bar, fit people avoid the thoughts of fat people as it relates to health and fitness. They have become desensitized to the middle-class mindset that once made them fat. Since all behavior begins with thought, fit people build relationships with other fit people to keep them moving in the right direction. Like the wealthy investor who ignores the ongoing hysteria and emotional rollercoaster of the financial markets, fit people ignore the excuses and victim mentality of fat people. The result is the same: The rich get richer, the fit get fitter, and the fat, fatter. The lesson is stop listening to people who are fat if you want to be fit. It's simple, but very few people seem to follow this age old advice.

Fat Loser Quote

    Fit people have learned to block out the opinions, beliefs and philosophies of the masses. Why follow the advice and example of people who are barely getting by? If your doctor is fat, get a new doctor. If your husband is a couch potato, stop listening to him about exercise. If your financial advisor is broke, trade him in for a rich one. The masses have been programmed and controlled for centuries by people of authority who were failing themselves. Fit people follow people who are more fit than they are, and they ignore everyone else in this area. They utilize this strategy in every area of their lives to get what they want.

Action Step

Stop listening to fat people who want to advise
you on how to get fit. Remember that most people
aren't very good at getting what they want.
Make a decision to only allow experts to guide
and influence you along your path to fitness.

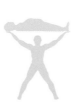

Fat people focus on the how

Fit people focus on the why

Middle-class thinkers imagine the life they desire and often quit before they start because they don't know how to make it reality. Linear thinking leads them to believe they have to know how to do something in order to make it happen. World-class thinkers know to ask for help if they don't understand how to do something, and go to work on figuring out why they should expend the effort. Diets are no different. Brilliant doctors and scientists have created the how-to part of the weight loss equation, but fat people still insist on questioning how their diets work. So while fat people wonder if the diet will work, fit people are searching for the emotional motivators that will keep them 100% compliant and moving forward when it gets tough. For some people 'the why' is to look and feel better. For others, it's a matter of life or death. Whatever the motivation, fit people know the secret is identifying what drives you and keeping it in front of you as much as possible. Emotional motivation is the power tool of the world class, yet it's barely understood at the lower levels of consciousness. It's so simple it's easy to underestimate, which is what many people do. When I lost 40 pounds in 12 weeks it wasn't because I was trying to get healthier, (although I'd love to say that) it was due almost entirely to an embarrassing situation where old friends didn't recognize me because I was so fat. I'm not proud of the fact that I was emotionally driven to lose weight by vanity, but it's true. Maybe it was shallow, but the bottom line is, it worked for me. I was used to getting compliments on my physique, and now people couldn't even recognize me because I'd gotten sloppy and allowed my body to become a grossly distorted version of itself. I was ashamed of my sloppy thinking and appearance, and holding that image of being embarrassed in my mind kept me going. Once you and your doctor have selected a healthy diet, keep reminding yourself why you're doing it. This one simple idea will make or break you.

Fat Loser Quote

❝ *Fat people get so engrossed in how they're going to get fit they miss the most important component of the process. Fit people designate the how-to of weight loss to the professionals who design diets and the doctors who recommend them. The great ones know their job is to develop a big enough reason to battle the bulge and win the weight loss war. Through a great deal of reflection and introspective thinking, they identify their emotional motivators that are driving them to get fit. They write their vision out on paper. They paste pictures of bodies they want to look like on poster boards. They focus their mental energy on bringing their dream body to life and keeping their attention on the pleasure and off the pain. While the masses are scouring every detail of their diet, the great ones are scouring every detail of the beautiful future they are on the road to inhabiting.* ❞

Critical Thinking Question

Are you aware that it's your emotional
motivators that will determine your
success or failure to get fit?

Action Step

Make a list of your five most powerful emotional
motivators for getting fit and read them every
morning. Stay connected to this list like scuba
diver does to oxygen. If you're emotional
motivation is unclear when the going gets
tough, your diet is in danger. Stay focused on
why you must get fit and remind yourself every
day as if you have no short term memory.
And always remember. . .You can do it!

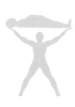

Afterword

Congratulations on being mentally tough enough to read this book all the way through! I'm aware of the preachy nature in which it was written. I know a lot of these philosophies sound judgmental, politically incorrect, shocking, and at times, even rude. All of this was for the purpose of waking you up to the reality that being fat is dangerous and needs to be addressed like any major threat to your life. I know at times you were thinking, 'God, this guy is a real jerk'. I thought the same thing! Some of the things I wrote even offended me! But I believe all human beings are spiritually connected, and I did it because I love you. The ferocity of my words is the manifestation of my burning desire to help you get fit and live the world-class life you deserve. I hope you'll forgive me for the manner in which I chose to express myself, but if my words have any impact on your success, it was worth it.

Thanks for reading this book.

Steve Siebold
December 17, 2008
Aspen, Colorado

Learning Resources

- *177 Mental Toughness Secrets*
  www.mentaltoughnesssecrets.com

- *177 Mental Toughness Secrets - CD Album*
  www.mentaltoughnesssecrets.com

- *Coaching 177 Mental Toughness Secrets*
  www.coachingmentaltoughness.com

- *Speaker Steve Siebold*
  www.speakerstevesiebold.com

- *Mental Toughness University*
  www.mentaltoughnessuniversity.com

- *Mental Toughness College*
  www.mentaltoughnesscollege.com

- *Mental Toughness Mastery*
  www.mentaltoughnessmastery.com

- *The Making of a Million Dollar Mind*
  www.milliondollarmind.com

- *Mental Toughness Institute for Weight Control*
  www.thefatlosers.com

- *Create The Future*
  www.networkmarketingleadership.com

- *John Maher, Painter of Speakers*
  www.painterofspeakers.com

- *Bill Gove Speech Workshop*
  www.feepaidprofessionalspeaker.com

- *Professional Speaker Show*
  www.professionalspeakershow.com

- *Siebold Success Network*
  www.sieboldsuccessnetwork.com

- *How To Market And Sell Yourself as a Professional Speaker*
  www.professionalspeakermarketing.com

- *Bill Gove Speech Club*
  www.billgovespeechclub.com

- *Bill Gove Speech Seminar*
  www.speechseminar.com

- *The Best Of Bill Gove*
  www.speechseminar.com

- *Speaking Is Easy . . . You Already Know How To Do It!*
  www.speakingeasy.com

- *The Ultimate Speaking Package*
  www.ultimatespeakingpackage.com

Do You Have What It Takes To Ascend To The Throne Of The World-Class?

Can a person of average intelligence and modest means ascend to the throne of the world class? 177 Mental Toughness Secrets of the World Class, identifies and explains the thought processes, habits, and philosophies of the world's greatest performers... and gives you action steps so you can implement these secrets immediately and get what you want.

People Who Adopt These 177 Mental Toughness Secrets Will Be Propelled To The Top. . .Both Personally And Professionally.

Here's What The World-Class is Saying About This Book:

"I find this book and Steve Siebold's mental toughness process to be life changing and liberating. I had a great personal and professional life before I was introduced to mental toughness. After three years of consecutive training, I have a superior life. Steve Siebold is the master of helping people prepare to win."

–Lou Wood
Region Business Director
Johnson & Johnson/OMP

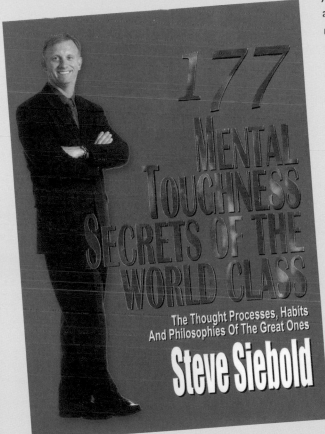

"If you're interested in jump-starting a journey of personal transformation, pick this book up and dive in anywhere. It's a treasure chest of compelling messages and practical exercises. It's up to you to do the work, but Steve Siebold will point you to all the right launching points."

– Amy Edmondson, Ph.D.
Professor of Business
Administration
Harvard Business School

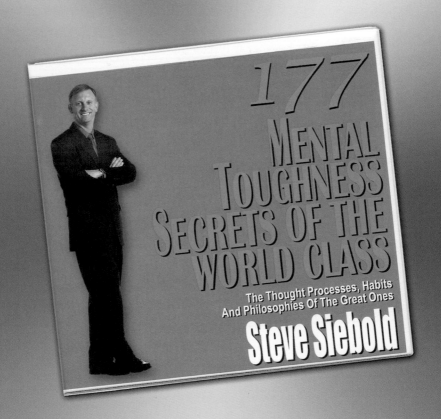

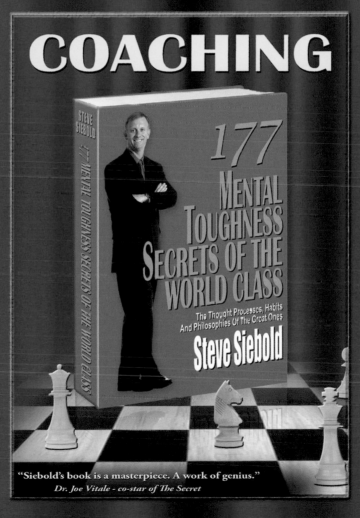

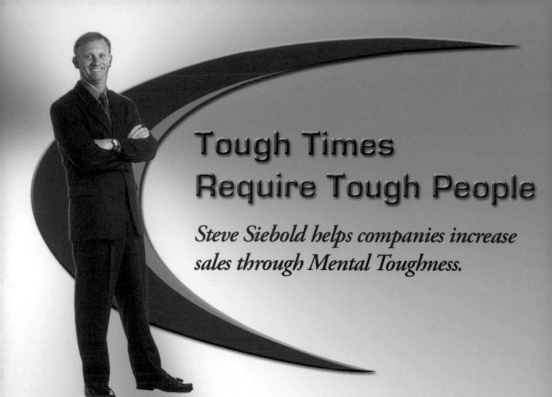

Tough Times
Require Tough People

Steve Siebold helps companies increase sales through Mental Toughness.

Steve will teach your people the secrets of the world-class... in a entertaining, enlightening way to increase their level of Mental Toughness.

If you're sales team is ready to take the mental toughness challenge, Steve Siebold is the speaker for your next meeting or convention.

See Steve delivering his keynote speech at a national convention in San Diego by visiting www.speakerstevesiebold.com or call 561-733-9078 for booking availability.

Steve Siebold, CSP, CPCS
www.speakerstevesiebold.com • 561-733-9078

Mental Toughness University
Helps Companies Increase Sales
And Move Market Share
By Creating A No Excuses-
High Performance Culture

Mental Toughness University is a comprehensive mental training process that moves sales and management teams from good to great. Mental Toughness trains people how to control their thoughts, feelings, and attitudes, before, during and after a performance. Especially under pressure.

What Are The Benefits of Mental Toughness Training?

Most MTU corporate clients are sales and management teams that report dramatic increases in sales. Management teams benefit by learning how to coach the mental toughness process and implement it immediately into their daily coaching with their sales team. Managers often adopt new criteria for hiring salespeople after completing the course. Employee retention rates are also affected due to the personal benefits gained during the training. MTU delivers both professional and personal results. Since most research shows that an employee's job is not the most important aspect of his or her life, the ongoing personal benefits of this program tend to raise the switching cost of an employee moving to another company. Companies often experience enhanced customer service from the participants as a result of their new level of focus on the customer.

Mental Toughness University is Not a Traditional Training Program.

MTU is a Process, Not a Program.

It's about training people how to THINK like world-class performers, and how to control and manipulate their own emotions for MAXIMUM performance. MTU is a cross between emotional intelligence training and critical thinking. It's an introspective process that causes people to examine their thoughts, feelings attitudes, and beliefs and how they are directly impacting their results. We call the process, 'Facilitated Introspection'. The six-hour program is an awakening to expose participants to the process and show them there's a higher level of emotional competence and mental performance than they are experiencing. MTU facilitates this emotional transformation over the next 12 months during the teleconference follow up program. Each participant is assigned 20 minutes of homework each week and held accountable for submitting it. Both the six-hour seminar and the follow-up teleconferences are highly interactive. Most people that go through the process have never been exposed to this level of personal introspection. They may be familiar with some of the content, but the real growth and change comes from them getting to know themselves. Most participants are shocked and surprised to learn how little they know about themselves. The Mental Toughness University Process has the power to bring out the best in any performer who will engage his or her mind in the process.

For more information, visit www.mentaltoughnessuniversity.com

Mental Toughness College

Building Million Dollar Minds.

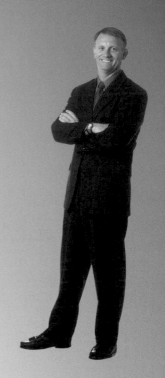

"Imagine doing what you want,

when you want, with whom you want,

for as long as you want, without

ever having to answer to anyone…"

That was my dream. My vision.

My ultimate fantasy . . .

. . . and it came true.

MENTAL TOUGHNESS MASTERY

12 CD Series

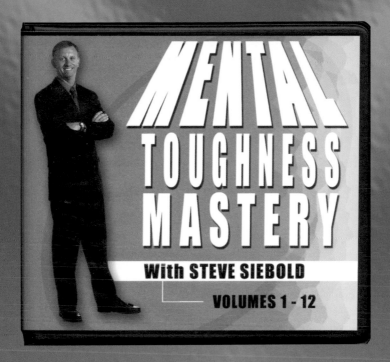

The great ones believe that nearly any goal is within their reach, and this single belief sets off a mental domino effect that continues to manifest one success after another. They literally THINK their way to the top, and 99% of them are no smarter than you and I.

Here's the problem:
It's not easy to make the distinction between the good and the great unless you know what you're looking for. After 20 years of studying champions, I've discovered that it's really a series of subtleties that add up to make the difference. Without knowing what to look for, most people will completely miss these subtleties. When you stand the champion next to a middle-class performer, there doesn't appear to be much difference. Have you ever thought to yourself, "I can't figure out why so and so is so successful; he/she doesn't seem to be any different than me or anyone else?"

Me, too. But not anymore. The differences are huge, but not very visible. So here's what I've done. I've selected the biggest differences between the winners and the still-trying, and I've put all of this information on a 12 CD series called Mental Toughness Mastery. You will receive 12 CDs detailing exactly how champions think and process information, as well as real life stories and examples of the world-class performers I've worked with over the years, and how to incorporate these ideas and philosophies into your life . . . immediately.

Order by calling 561.733.9078 or visit www.mentaltoughnessmastery.com

The Making Of A
Million Dollar Mind

"Have You Got What It Takes To Produce Million Dollar Results?"

For most people, the answer is YES and NO.

YES, they have the POTENTIAL and TALENT.

NO, they lack the BELIEF SYSTEM it takes to ACHIEVE and SUSTAIN World Class Results.

It's sad, but true.

That's why you see people who have won the lottery losing it, or getting in trouble with the IRS, or plagued with other self-induced difficulties.

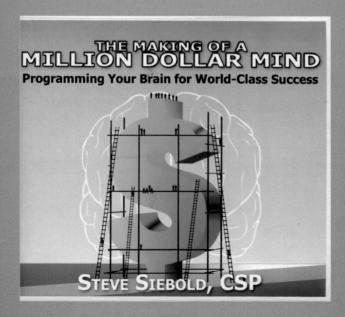

For the top ten distinctions between middle class and world class thinkers visit

www.milliondollarmind.com

MENTAL TOUGHNESS INSTITUTE FOR WEIGHT CONTROL

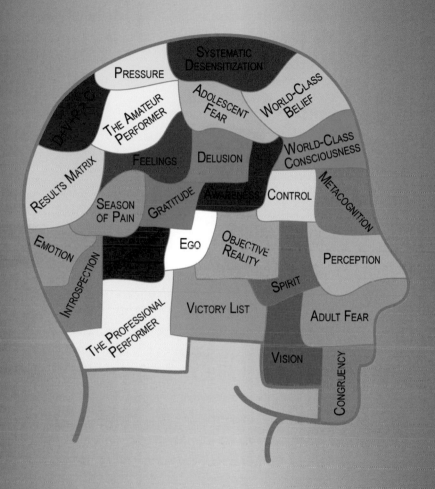

MTI is a mental toughness training and support system designed to work in conjuntion with your diet and exercise program. It's a 12-week telecourse that combines mental toughness training with a national support network. It's a cross between a support group and boot camp!

CREATE THE FUTURE

MP3 Download

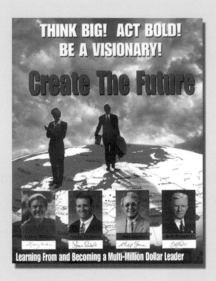

Your multi-million dollar leadership team consists of Bob Proctor, the master of income acceleration . . . Larry Wilson, leadership guru of the Fortune 500 . . . Bill Gove, the father of professional speaking . . . and Steve Siebold, mental toughness trainer of champions.

In this ground-breaking program, these world-renowned experts teach you how to apply the secrets that catapulted them to the pinnacle of their professions – and how YOU can apply their collective wisdom to dramatically accelerate the growth of your network marketing business.

Never in the history of network marketing have leaders of this magnitude joined forces to share their secrets of success – and give YOU the tools necessary to create your future and become a multi-million dollar leader in the field of network marketing.

**Order by calling 561.733.9078 or visit
www.networkmarketingleadership.com**

Thomas Kinkade
is the Painter of Light...

Peter Max
is the Painter of Pop Art...

John Maher
is the Painter of Public Speakers

John Maher
Celebrates the Life and Legacy of

Bill Gove,
the Father of Professional Speaking

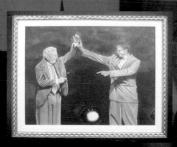

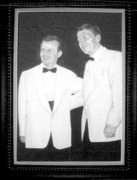

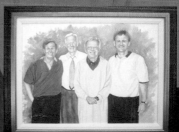

www.painterofspeakers.com

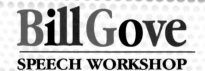

Professional Speaker Show

The Art and Business of Professional Public Speaking

Listen to Steve Siebold, CSP
On How You Can Become A Professional Speaker!

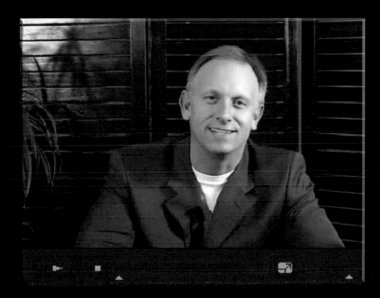

24/7 ACCESS
TO INSIDE INFORMATION ABOUT
PROFESSIONAL SPEAKING

Professional Speaker Show.com

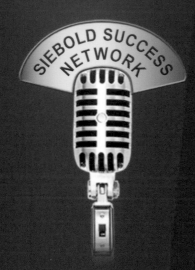

How To Market And Sell Yourself As A Professional Speaker:

The truth about what it REALLY takes to make it in the professional speaking business.

If you have ever considered a professional speaking career, this may be the beginning of a very successful, fulfilling, financially rewarding journey. How to Market and Sell Yourself as a Professional Speaker debunks the myths and mysteries of the professional speaking business, and reveals the truth and little known behind the scenes information that only an insider can give you. Nothing is held back on this album. You won't hear any hype or rah-rah nonsense...just the facts about how to succeed in the speaking business at the six and seven-figure level.

Some of the things you will learn:

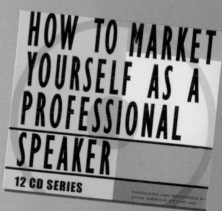

- How to select the right topic and connect it to solving a problem that individuals and organizations will pay for

- How to market and sell yourself to major corporations for substantial fees

- How to set your speaking fees based on your speaking skills and value proposition

- How to market to the 400 major speakers bureaus

- How to create a multidimensional marketing machine for your speaking business

- How to gain national recognition as a topical expert by writing articles and columns for magazines and trade journals

- How to create CD and DVD albums that make money while you sleep

- How to conduct, market and sell hundreds of thousands of dollars in training over the telephone with less than 2% overhead

- How to conduct, market and sell your own international private coaching program in person or over the telephone

- How to create ongoing lead generation systems for your speeches, seminars, workshops, coaching programs, consulting services and CD, tape, and video albums

For more information, visit www.professionalspeakermarketing.com

Where Do Executives, Professionals, Celebrities And Professional Speakers PRACTICE Their Speaking Skills And TEST Their Material?

The Bill Gove Speech Club

The BGSC is an international network of exclusive professional public speaking clubs for advanced speakers. Since 1947 the Bill Gove Speech Workshop has been known as the Harvard of Professional Speaking Schools, training more world-class speakers than any organization in history.

Are You Ready To Join Us?

Bill Gove
SPEECH CLUB

New York City	St. Louis	Scottsdale	Vancouver
Los Angeles	Minneapolis	Detroit	Montreal
Philadelphia	Denver	El Paso	Johannesburg
Washington DC	Palm Beach	Portland	Cape Town
Phoenix	Ft. Lauderdale	Milwaukee	London
Dallas	Aspen	Tampa	Paris
Houston	Louisville	Toronto	Edinburgh
Atlanta	Albuquerque	Halifax	Sydney
Chicago	San Francisco	Calgary	Melbourne
Boston			Brisbane

www.billgovespeechclub.com

Imagine...

Gaining Over A Half-Century Of Wisdom In Professional Speaking Skills In Just 6 Hours... In The Privacy Of Your Own Home... Direct From The Most Successful Professional Speaking School In The World.

What you will learn

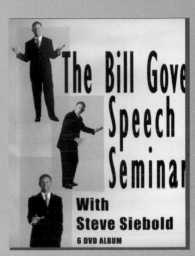

- How to write and catalog speeches like a professional speaker
- The secret of the world's best speakers
- The support secret that professional speakers use to relax before every speech
- How to use theatrical techniques in your presentation
- The grand prix racing vocalization technique
- How to integrate humor into any speech. What to do if you go blank on stage
- The pressure-proofing system that will end stage fright...forever
- How to create your speeches with passion...but deliver them with skill
- The two tools you must own to develop your skills
- The Mark Twain technique of handcrafting every speech

This six DVD set is loaded with so much content you will have to view it numerous times to digest it all. Learn fifty years of the best speaking and speech writing skills in the profession.

If you're serious about public speaking or building a career as a fee paid professional speaker, this may be the opportunity you've been looking for. Sixty years of information on six DVD's.

It would take you YEARS to learn all of this material by trial and error...or you could simply invest in this program and learn it over the course of a couple of days, and have it on DVD to be able to review over and over again.

For more information visit www.speechseminar.com

THE BEST OF BILL GOVE

MP3 Download

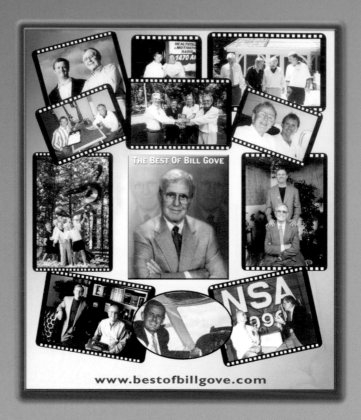

www.bestofbillgove.com

Listen, Laugh and Learn with one of the most celebrated professional speakers and philosophers of all-time: Mr. Bill Gove. This series captures Bill Gove at the most magical times of his 54-year speaking career. From his famous 1954 sales speech for 13,000 people at the International Amphitheatre in Chicago ... to his 1991 Golden Gavel Acceptance Speech in Atlanta. These speeches are the heart and soul of Bill Gove's philosophies on business, love, life and living. You'll never see the world the same way after you've seen it through the eyes of Bill Gove.

Bill Gove, CSP, CPAE 1912-2001

Bill Gove was known around the world as the Father of the Professional Speaking Industry. He was the first President of the National Speakers Association, and one of the most popular speakers of the 20th century. He was inducted into the International Speakers Hall of Fame in 1975, and honored as the International Speaker of the Year in 1976. Mr. Gove won the Cavett Award in 1980, (The Oscar of Professional Speaking) and Toastmasters International's Golden Gavel Award in 1991. In 1997, he partnered with Steve Siebold to from the Gove Siebold Group, an international training and consulting firm based in Boynton Beach, Florida.

Order by calling 561.733.9078 or visit www.bestofbillgove.com

SPEAKING IS EASY . . .

YOU ALREADY KNOW HOW TO DO IT!

By Steve Siebold & Bill Gove

MP3 Download

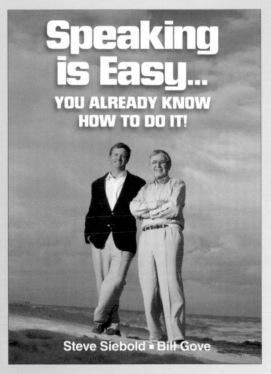

This downloadable MP3 explains the world-famous PowerBoard system direct from the vault of the Bill Gove Speech Workshop. This is your only opportunity to hear the PowerBoard system explained by the great Bill Gove himself; because it was the only recording he ever made detailing the system. You'll hear live speeches, Bill Gove made in sold-out auditoriums around the United States during the 1960s, 70s, 80s and 90s. These speeches will give you a great feel for what goes into to the making of a world-class speech, and how you can adapt and upgrade your content and speaking style to do the same. This album is super-informative and highly entertaining. After you listen to it, you'll know exactly why Bill Gove was regarded as the master of masters on the platform.

Order by calling 561.733.9078 or visit www.speakingeasy.com

THE ULTIMATE SPEAKING PACKAGE

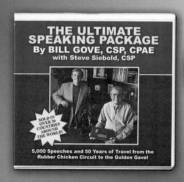

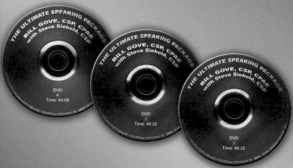

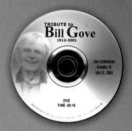

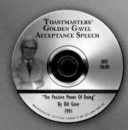

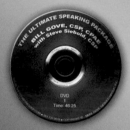

The Ultimate Speaking Package is for serious and aspiring speakers who want the very best information ever assembled on public speaking . . . at a VIP price.

The package includes:

Everything You Need To Know About Speaking, by Bill Gove. This 4 DVD album is an exclusive 3 hour fireside chat with the father of professional speaking, Mr. Bill Gove. Bill offers the tips, techniques, and speaking strategies that made him one of the most popular professional speakers of the 20th century. This is a behind the scenes, backstage interview with the master of masters, telling it like it was and like it is in the world of professional speaking. The stories Bill tells on these videos are worth their weight in gold. This one of a kind album is a classic and a must have in your personal library. It's been sold in 30 countries around the world.

The Tribute to Bill Gove: A Celebration of the Father of Professional Speaking (1 hour DVD) Bill Gove passed away on December 9, 2001. On July 17, 2002, 250 of the greatest speakers in the world gathered in Orlando, Florida to pay tribute to the man and the legend. Bill Gove Speech Workshop graduates Dave Yoho Sr. and Steve Siebold emceed this event that included comments by Zig Ziglar, Larry Wilson, and Don Hutson. It also includes excerpts of Bill Gove speaking in 1967, 1973, 1991, and his final speech on September 25, 2001.

**Order by calling 561.733.9078 or visit
www.ultimatespeakingpackage.com**

About the Author

Steve Siebold, CSP, CPCS, is an internationally recognized expert in the field of mental toughness training. His Fortune 500 clients include Johnson & Johnson, Procter & Gamble, GlaxoSmithKline, Toyota and Harrah's Entertainment. His first book, *177 Mental Toughness Secrets of the World Class*, sold over 100,000 copies. As a professional speaker, Steve addresses approximately 60 live audiences per year and ranks among the top 1% of income earners worldwide. In 2007, Steve won the prestigious Telly Award for most outstanding host for his national television show, *Mental Toughness of Champions*. In 2009, he co-starred in the feature film, *Beyond the Secret*, the long awaited follow up to the mega-hit movie, The Secret, which was seen by over 1 billion people worldwide.

Steve resides in Palm Beach County, Florida and Lake Lanier, Georgia, with wife Dawn and family animals Robin the rat dog and sugar gliders Einstein and Maslow.